Woody

Woody

BARBARA SHELTON
with BOB TERRELL

CHRISTIAN HERALD BOOKS
Chappaqua, New York

Library of Congress Cataloging in Publication Data

Shelton, Barbara.
  Woody.

  1. Amyotrophic lateral sclerosis—Biography.   2. Shelton, Elwood, 1926–1975.   3. Christian life—1960-   I. Terrell, Bob, joint author.   II. Title.
RC406.A24S53   248'.86'0924   79-50949
ISBN 0-915684-52-7

CHRISTIAN HERALD BOOKS, 40 Overlook Drive, Chappaqua, New York 10514.

Manufactured in the United States of America.

To
our son Dan,
who stood beside us through it all

INTRODUCTION

My husband, Woody, dying slowly for several years, endured that portion of his life with dignity. Out of his suffering, a great richness came to him and to many around him.

He is happy now, finally at peace, and he still lives in the hearts of those who loved him.

I learned many things during his illness. Among them were: never say no to God; never say no to your problems; and, most emphatically, never say no to a dying man.

Barbara Shelton
Hendersonville,
North Carolina
July 29, 1978

1

Softly, during the night, the snow fell—big, beautiful flakes that clung to the evergreens and the bare oak branches.

I didn't know that it had snowed. I had been so exhausted the previous evening from long weeks of day and night caring for Woody that our son Dan insisted I go home and sleep. It was Saturday night, and our night nurse was off. Dan asked a friend who was a nurse to stay with him, just to keep him awake, and I slept as he worked through the night with his father.

At 7:30 Sunday morning, November 23, 1975, the telephone rang. I jumped from bed immediately. It had to be Dan.

"Mom," Dan said, "I think you'd better come back to the hospital now."

I knew that Woody was dead.

"All right," I said. "I'll come immediately."

"No," Dan's voice was firm. "I'm sending Dale for you." Dale was our friend.

"I'm all right," I said. "I can drive."

"Mom, you don't understand," Dan said. "There is the most beautiful snow I've ever seen."

Anticipating a quick trip to the hospital, I had laid out my clothes the night before, underclothing, skirt, blouse. I pulled back the drapes and looked out upon a white wonderland. The snow lay so softly and quietly. Everything was hushed. I went to the closet and added boots and my warmest coat to the things I intended to wear.

I had known the night before that Woody would die soon. As I drove home, the feeling that I would never see him alive again was almost overpowering. Yet I had slept peacefully. I knew in my heart that I had done everything possible for Woody. The moment I left the hospital, the feeling of his imminent death had come over me, and I could find nothing in my heart to regret: I had given Woody all my time these last two years.

We had all lost our fear of death—Woody, Dan, and myself. After he lost control of his muscular and nervous systems, his frail body began to wither, and we had begun to look forward to the release of death; we had even wished for it.

These thoughts ran through my mind as I dressed. Soon there was a knock at the back door. Dale's hands were shoved into the pockets of his wool jacket.

"Barbara," he said, "are you ready to go?" His voice was quiet and kind, and very gentle.

As he drove through the four-inch snow, I marveled at the beauty of God's handiwork. I had only half-combed my hair, just brushed it back, and wore no makeup, but it didn't matter.

We walked up the back stairway of the hospital to the second floor, a route that was thoroughly familiar. I pushed open the door to Woody's room. All the nurses in that unit were gathered around Woody's bed, and they had tears in their eyes.

The bed was raised high, and Woody lay on it, unmoving. His eyes were still open, though he was dead,

and as I walked across the room his eyes seemed to fol-
low me like the eyes in a beautiful portrait that seem to
focus upon you regardless of where you are. Even as I
approached the bed, his eyes stayed upon me.

Dan stood on the other side of the bed. Beside him
was the nurse who had kept him awake through the
night. There had been little else she could do because of
the problem of communicating with Woody.

I took Woody's hand in my left hand and placed my
right hand on his shoulder. He looked peaceful. His face
was calm after the many months of severe mental and
physical torture. There was a hint of contentment in his
features now.

"Woody," I said, "you can't believe it, there's the most
beautiful snow I've ever seen."

It seldom snows in Hendersonville, North Carolina, in
November. I looked out the window. This would have
been Woody's day for deer hunting with Dr. Bill
Lampley and his friends, Buddy Richardson, Frank
Drake, Al Geremonte, and Bill Waggoner. Woody had
gone instead to a different place, a special place.

I talked to Woody and told him how beautiful it was
outside. "You know that God has painted the most magnificent picture just for you," I told him, "a special day,
and a special performance, to take you to a very special
place."

The nurses' tears were flowing freely now, but neither
Dan nor I could cry. We knew in our hearts that Woody
had lived each day to the fullest. Only the last two or
three years had been filled with suffering and pain. The
rest had been beauty and contentment, doing the things
he loved to do, enjoying the experiences of a good life-
time.

Now he had journeyed through the Valley of the
Shadow. Superficially, it appeared that Woody was the

loser, but I felt that it was the other way around. At that moment, I felt that somewhere Woody was free of this troubled world, free of his pain, and that he walked and talked and felt and loved and was happy.

I looked into his face, and a thought of tremendous proportions came over me. Woody, you have seen God!

I looked at each person in the room, and thought how we all would continue to live with the pain and problems of life. Then I looked back at Woody's body lying in yellow nylon pajamas on the taut, white sheet, a body that weighed only eighty pounds, less than half his weight two years ago, and I knew that because of Woody, we— Dan and I, at least—would be able to handle the problems and pain, for Woody had touched our lives in a special way. We would never be the same.

Woody had been stricken by a dreaded illness, and as he lay in his hospital bed, God had enriched our lives. He had given us a great understanding of caring for those who are ill and in need of help or love. He had made us see the beautiful things of life each day. He had taught us to appreciate speech and love for each other, and he had showed us that we shouldn't take our many freedoms for granted.

We stood around the bed talking for several minutes. Dan told how, during the night, the snow had come down, and how peaceful it had been in the room as he turned his father periodically and worked with him. Woody had been coherent until the last few hours.

As Dan talked, I glanced around the room. I had already removed many things, knowing the end was near. As I left the hospital those last few days, I carried home flowers, clothes, and things we had accumulated over a period of months. The hospital room was so large and nice, almost like a suite, that we had practically made a home there.

I didn't feel Woody's presence in the room anymore.

Dr. Lampley came in. He examined Woody and pronounced him dead. Then he put his arm around me.

"Let's go," he said.

"I'll stay and clean the room," I said.

"No, you've done enough," he said. "Others will clean the room."

Dan came around the bed, and Dr. Lampley led us out of the room and down the hall to a little waiting room by the nurses' station. We sat and talked, and I filled out the necessary forms and release papers. My father and my brother Leon came in.

As we talked in the waiting room, furnished with a few chairs, a table, a lamp, and dirty ashtrays not yet cleaned, I noticed that neither Dr. Lampley nor my brother had shaved and that my father had hurriedly dressed; but it didn't matter. The important thing that morning was our flow of thoughts, and to talk and share.

Dan and I shared feelings of peace and joy in our hearts that Woody was finally released after many months in a prison of suffering. His disease was known as amyotrophic lateral sclerosis, or "Lou Gehrig's disease," an illness the medical world is still quite helpless to treat.

We had been through a period of tremendous challenge, a growth period we would never forget. We thought it amazing how we were blessed through such a traumatic experience. We had felt the presence of God with us each day, and he had shown us that by living one day at a time we could cope. Things seemed easier to accept on a daily basis. Early on, God had promised that he would be with us through it all, and we had found this to be true. We had only to believe.

Now we thanked the nurses for their kindnesses to us, and Dan drove me home. My father and Leon and Dale followed.

They cleaned the snow from the walk because they

knew friends would come. I busied myself straightening things around the house, and soon the phone and the doorbell began to ring.

The house filled quickly with neighbors and friends who told us they loved us. They had come to share our sorrow and loss. Woody had touched their lives, too.

The day warmed, and by early afternoon the snow had disappeared. It was evident, I thought, that God had made a special performance just for Woody, who loved snow and who could hardly contain himself to stay inside when snowflakes began to fall.

The next day was filled making funeral arrangements. Dan, Woody's brother Raymond, and I drove to the mortuary to make final plans, and that evening we received friends and relatives.

I had thought of several places to put Woody, and finally decided on a little country cemetery. It was open and free, and he loved the outdoors so much I knew he would have liked it. The cemetery was at the back of a small country church—the Tracy Grove Wesleyan Methodist—where we had attended.

We asked Reverend Stanley not to say anything about Woody because we felt his life spoke for itself. Nothing could be said to change it in any way.

At the service, the organist played "How Great Thou Art," and Mr. Stanley read from the Bible. One verse, Micah 6:8, stood out above all others: "He hath showed thee, O man, what is good; and what doth the Lord require of thee, but to do justly, and to love mercy, and to walk humbly with thy God?" Except for a brief, two-year period in his life, that verse described Woody. The rest of the service was simple, yet beautiful, and appropriate for Woody.

After the service, we walked to the back of the church where Woody was buried. The cemeterey was quiet and peaceful—and cold. Suddenly I began to chill, and my whole body shook. Next to me, Dan was also shaking.

The casket was lowered into the grave, and we turned away. We would never see Woody again on earth.

We had been through a period of life that most people never experience, and we had learned. We had loved, we had cared, and we knew that because of Woody and his Trojanlike battle against the incurable disease, our lives could be meaningful to others.

A verse of Scripture came to me then, 2 Cor. 1:3-4: "Blessed be God . . . who comforteth us in all our tribulation, that we may be able to comfort them which are in any trouble, by the comfort wherewith we ourselves are comforted of God."

We felt God's presence, and we were determined that Woody had not died in vain. I decided then and there to write this book.

2

The afternoon of October 6, 1973 was one of those bright, golden days in the mountains of North Carolina. The trees were turning to red, orange, yellow, vermillion, rust, and gold, and were within a week of reaching their color peak.

Although a beautiful day outside, inside the office of Dr. Phillip Sellers in Hendersonville things were less than bright.

"Barbara," he said, and there was a hesitancy in his voice, "I hate to tell you this, but I have found that Woody has a very rare illness called amyotrophic lateral sclerosis. It is more commonly known as Lou Gehrig's disease. . . ."

Lou Gehrig's disease!

I had feared the worst—and this was it. I had read about Lou Gehrig, the famous team captain of the New York Yankees, the pride of the baseball world, struck down in the prime of life by this dread disease, withered and dead at the age of 38. . . .

"The illness," Dr. Sellers said, "is sometimes called the 'killer disease.' Unfortunately, there is no known cure. It is progressive with or without treatment. There is nothing we can do professionally to help him, except to make him as comfortable as possible."

Dr. Sellers was gentle, though he minced no words. I felt a shock run through my body. Killer disease . . . no known cure . . . nothing we can do. . . .

"Therapy trials," he said, "have been conducted in various neurological centers with a number of drugs—neostigmine, isoprinosine, guanidine, the cortcosteroids—but published reports on these and others are not encouraging.

"The life span is from one to three years—five at the most—except in a few extreme cases where the illness arrested itself. There is a possibility he will lose the use of all his extremities. Some patients reach a point where they are unable to hold up their heads. As a rule, they have difficulty swallowing, and they can lose their speech entirely."

The only nondiscouraging thing he told me was, "Through the illness, Woody's mind will remain coherent. ALS victims know everyone and everything; they experience pain and other sensations of the body, but they become unable to move, unable to help themselves. Sight and hearing are usually not affected."

He told me more concerning the illness, all the while emphasizing that the whole medical profession knew little about ALS since it was extremely rare.

There had not been any breakthrough in research, and it appeared to be totally up to me to learn to cope with the disease. The doctor assured me it made no difference where I took Woody, that no one could do anything about curing him.

It seemed as though he was telling me a story about someone I didn't know. I thanked him and left his office with the strangest feeling in my body, almost as if I were suddenly living in a different world.

I didn't realize just how different my world would become.

I remember checking with the nurse at the desk, leaving the office, and getting into my car. I was aware of people around me, but I didn't know who they were. I didn't even notice the golden trees. I have no recollection of how long I sat in the car with thoughts and memories flooding my mind.

3

Woody was born in Olive Hill, Kentucky, on June 4, 1926, the son of a traveling minister who christened him Elwood Shelton. His father was on the road most of the time, traveling to remote parts of Kentucky and surrounding states, preaching wherever he could.

When he was eight, Woody lost his mother. Nine months pregnant, she fell down a flight of stairs. With no doctor available, and only a midwife in attendance, she died. But before death, she gave birth to a perfectly healthy baby girl.

Losing his mother at such an early age transformed Woody's life. Her ability to produce his baby sister, Ines, before she died made an indelible impression on Woody.

The Sheltons lived in a frame house overlooking the brickyards in Olive Hill. The kilns were among the largest in the country, and millions of clay bricks were fired there. Woody spent hours watching the valley where the enormous fires glowed.

Mountain folk lived there. Many were self-sufficient types who said that money wasn't everything. All they needed was enough to pay taxes and buy staples for their tables. They were willing to make do or do without.

Woody Shelton knew at an early age that he didn't want to live that kind of life. He dreamed of faraway places, constantly wondering when and how he would leave Olive Hill and see the world.

He worked after school and on weekends bagging groceries and doing odd jobs in the grocery store. Olive Hill was a rough place. Once, as Woody swept the street in front of the grocery, the police had a shootout with an outlaw across the street. The mortally wounded brigand fell dead before Woody's eyes.

Every weekend, against his father's wishes, Woody slipped into town to see Tom Mix movies. The elder Shelton was a fire-and-brimstone fundamentalist preacher who believed that movies were evil. He was the strictest sort of man. Every time the church doors were opened, Woody and his friends were required by their parents to attend.

Woody and his friends would also go across town and sit outside the Church of God, listening to the tuneful singing, shouting, and talking in tongues. They didn't understand it, but they were quite fascinated by this religion that was strange to their upbringing.

Woody spent his summers fishing, swimming, hunting, and picnicking with the family. He and his friends caught squirrels. Often the Shelton family had squirrel for Thanksgiving, and occasionally they ate squirrel for Christmas dinner.

"Pop always said the blessing," Woody said, "always sat at the head of the table, and always helped his plate first."

Dorothy, the oldest child, mothered her brothers and sisters, working hard to keep the family together, but one by one they drifted their separate ways. "We loved Dorothy dearly," Woody said. "She was the only mother I ever really knew."

Woody played football, basketball, and baseball in high school and excelled in each. He also studied hard and made good grades, but since there was little money in the family—and no way to make any real money—he was unable to go to college when he graduated from high school.

On a Saturday afternoon in January 1944, with America fighting a feverish war with the Germans and Japanese, Woody packed a small bag, caught the bus to Cincinnati, and joined the navy. Finally, he was off to see the world, never to return to Olive Hill more than a half-dozen times, and these for only short visits.

The world that Woody Shelton saw was the Atlantic Ocean. He saw it from on board the U.S.S. *Baker*, a destroyer escort. But World War II wasn't the only war that Woody fought: he also fought one within himself, trying to fashion a trade that would earn a livelihood.

Woody learned to box. He was a featherweight, and he learned the trade well. Always athletic, he soon racked up a string of victories that attracted the attention of all aboard the U.S.S. *Baker*.

There were other battles as well. Off Gibraltar, the *Baker* sank a German submarine filled with 15- to 17-year-old boys, and this tore at the strings of Woody's tender heart.

He was so tenderhearted that it was a wonder he excelled in boxing. He had a deep compassion and understanding for others, and he could never offend anyone. Woody scored knockouts in the ring with a right hook that was almost apologetic.

But he was determined. He fought well.

4

Woody left the navy in 1946 and continued to box. He was a middleweight, about 160 pounds, and occasionally fought as a light heavyweight. His father had remarried and still lived in Olive Hill, but Woody was not inclined to return there. He knew his father would frown on his pugilistic career.

His fighting took him all over the eastern United States, from Pennsylvania and Ohio to Florida. He moved to Hendersonville for several good reasons. It was centrally located, and the fresh mountain air was conducive to good training. Jack Dempsey had trained in Hendersonville for his second fight with Gene Tunney. Also, his brother Raymond, who was a Methodist minister, lived with his family in Hendersonville, and Woody could live with them.

Woody bought a big Harley-Davidson motorcycle on which he cruised the mountain roads. He worked hard, trained well, and became something of a playboy. Boxers, then, were glamorous figures—if they were winners, which Woody Shelton was.

He came into my life on a hot, muggy afternoon in the summer of 1949. I went to a skating party with a local guy who was nice, but nothing special. As we skated the afternoon away, I kept noticing a very handsome young man doing all kinds of figure eights. He was light on his feet and easy on the skates. He flitted about with the great confidence of one who knows exactly what he is doing.

He was about five-feet-eight, 160 pounds, trim and well-built, and I judged him to be about 18. I was only 15. He was with an attractive young girl, but he paid less attention to her than to his skating. I thought him extremely good looking; he had dark, wavy hair, a sort of baby face, and a fantastically smooth complexion. I had no idea that he was a boxer; his face was unmarked, but his muscles bulged beneath his tight-fitting shirt and he was obviously athletic.

Each time he circled the floor, he came closer and closer to me. The young man I was with kept watching him and saying, "Who does he think he is?" I watched him, too, and wondered the same thing, though with a different degree of emotion. My date became uncomfortable and irritated as the muscular young man paid attention to me.

Suddenly, in the crowded confusion, someone crashed into my back, and I splattered all over the floor. I tried to get up, and a sharp pain shot through my right foot. I thought I had broken my foot.

My date was confused. He wanted to call an ambulance, or at least get a stretcher for me. When he went to look for one, this handsome guy appeared from nowhere, and with his strong arms picked me up as if I were a pillow. He carried me the long way around the rink to the lounge.

He removed my skates and began massaging my foot and ankle. I melted on the chair! Before my date found me, I was up and walking, though limping from the sprain, and I knew my foot was not broken.

I thanked the young man, who said his name was

Woody Shelton, and we went separate ways. I hoped that would not be the last time I saw him.

The next day, Sunday, I went to church, and when I got home, the phone was ringing. I answered and immediately recognized Woody's voice.

"Hello, Barbara," he said. "This is Woody. How are you feeling?"

His call so surprised me that I struggled for words, and finally muttered, "I'm fine."

"Could I come by today?" he asked. "I'd like to see you."

"Sure," I said, thrilled to my toenails.

I watched the road until he drove up in a 1941 Ford. He wore a light blue knit shirt and dark blue slacks. He looked absolutely great!

I wore a skirt halfway to my ankles, bobby socks, and white saddle oxfords. When I think about it now, I have to laugh. I must have looked like I was wearing greaves around my legs, but those were the fashions of the day.

We sat in the living room and talked all afternoon, covering everything except his age. I asked how old he was, and he evaded the question, or joked that he was "old enough," or simply changed the subject. I'm sure he was afraid that if he admitted he was 23, eight years older than I, that I wouldn't see him any more.

When I finally found out, it was too late. I was hopelessly in love with him.

On September 1, 1950, we were married, and that was one of the proudest moments of my life.

5

Because of me, Woody sold his motorcycle and stopped boxing. I couldn't stand to see anyone hurt, especially him, and I was afraid of both his profession and his toy. I had heard of people being torn to pieces in motorcycle wrecks, and I didn't want it to happen to him. We had no words over these things; he simply gave them up because he knew I feared them. I didn't want to lose a good friend and husband.

I never saw him box, but friends said he was good. He might have stayed with it if he had thought he was good enough to get into the championship class, but he had enough sense to know he could make a living without getting his brains beaten out in club fights.

Woody was a real sportsman in every respect. He loved everything about the Great Outdoors and had a wonderfully earthy way of living. He teased me because I had to know what made everything tick. He said I was too much of a perfectionist.

We were different, yet much alike. I was an extrovert, he an introvert. When we were married, I had no particular liking for hunting and fishing, but I decided early in our marriage that if I wanted to be with him, I would have to learn. With or without me, he would hunt and fish. It wasn't that he didn't love me, it was just that he loved the outdoors so much.

Woody was good. He caught fish where no one else did. I learned as much as I could about fishing. I got to the point finally where I could bait my own hook, but I couldn't have learned to fish like Woody in two life-times.

Woody was also an excellent marksman, and while I never became adept at stalking game and getting in that telling shot, I did learn to cook all sorts of meat, and Woody kept us supplied with venison and small game.

The wild food came in handy, too. We rented a small apartment on the west side of Hendersonville, and Woody managed a cut-rate gas station. He didn't make a lot of money, so his hunting and fishing helped with the grocery bills.

Since he had to work long hours and sometimes far into the night, I was alone too much. We decided to move to the country and live with my family so the nights wouldn't be as lonely, and I would be safe. Woody worried about working nights and leaving me at home alone.

Early in 1951, we discovered that I was pregnant, and on August 30, just two days before our first wedding an-niversary, I gave birth to a premature baby boy. We named him Daniel Lee. He weighed three pounds, seven ounces, and had to stay in the hospital for several weeks.

Oddly enough, Danny's early birth was brought on by the same accident that had cost Woody's mother her life. I fell down a flight of stairs. Thank God, there were doc-tors nearby to care for me, or I, too, might have died in childbirth.

Danny remained in an oxygen tent in the hospital for six weeks before I was given permission to hold him. How my arms ached for him! He was so small we carried him on a pillow for months, but we thought he was the most beautiful child we had ever seen. When we went shopping, people stopped me on the streets and in the stores to talk to him. He loved all the attention and developed a fantastic personality.

Danny grew quite rapidly, and within a year he was an average, healthy lad.

We saved our money and bought a small lot on Lake Lure, near Chimney Rock. It was a beautiful place. We built a boathouse and made plans to build a cabin, a retreat where we could get away from town and enjoy the outdoors on weekends.

Woody left the gas station and went to work for his friend, Buddy Richardson, who owned a paint store. He enjoyed the work and soon rose to the position of office manager. I got a job as an assistant to Dr. Leonard Barber, a fine dentist who did complete dental reconstructions.

Lake Lure was only twenty miles from home, and when Woody and I came home from work in the summertime, when the days were longer, we would take Danny and drive to Lake Lure and water ski until dark. We all learned to ski quite well. Of course, we spent weekends there as well.

We prospered. We never got far enough ahead to be classed as wealthy, or even well-off, but we saved enough money to build the cabin at Lake Lure.

We slept under the stars on top of the boathouse until we built the cabin. Rather, Woody and Danny slept—I always managed to see the moon come up, cross the sky, and go down. At one time, I thought I could tell you how many stars were in the heavens. For some reason, I was never comfortable sleeping outside, but Woody and Danny loved it. They could have continued forever.

Fortunately for me, we managed to build the cabin before too long, and then we became normal people once again, sleeping indoors like most others who weekended at the lake. Still, Woody and Danny occasionally took their sleeping bags and spent the night on top of the boathouse.

Sometimes Woody and Danny went on fishing trips to Lake Hartwell in South Carolina, a sprawling lake in the upper part of the state. Both were expert fishermen and kept us well supplied with fish.

Danny filled out as the years passed and grew quite strong. Like his father, he developed a tremendous love for the outdoors.

Around the first of November each year, Woody would take his .30-06 down from the gun rack and clean and polish it until you could see your reflection in the stock. We thought it was made of precious metal; Woody thought it to be pure gold.

Nothing stood in the way of his deer hunting. We knew that November—the deer season—was his month. I kidded him about that. I often told him that if I died in November, they'd have to wait till December to bury me.

He would laugh and say, "You're right. How did you guess?" In his own special way, he loved to kid me.

Woody had never been ill in his life, except for the flu and a few minor sicknesses. He was, as he said, healthy as a horse. Who would suspect that a man like him would ever be felled by something as terrible as amyotrophic lateral sclerosis?

Danny progressed through kindergarten, grammar school, and junior high. He had all the usual childhood diseases, but nothing more. At the start of his sophomore year in high school, we sent him off to a private religious school in eastern North Carolina. He made good grades through the school year, liked the new friends he made, came home for the summer, and made plans to return in the fall.

On a Sunday afternoon that summer, we were water skiing on Lake Lure. Danny was out on the skis, Woody drove the boat, and I sat in the back, enjoying the warmth of the afternoon and the companionship of the men I loved.

Suddenly, a big boat loomed up behind Danny, flying across the water at a much higher speed than we were going. I screamed to Danny, but as the boat flashed past him, lifting him on the edge of its wake, he lost his balance and fell into the water. His lower right side struck the ski.

We fished him out of the lake and went immediately to the cabin. All afternoon he was in pain, and he chilled most of the night, but did not want us to call a doctor.

"I'll be all right," he said repeatedly.

But the next day he was unable to stand, and the pain in the lower part of his back was excruciating. He was ready then to see a doctor.

For a week the doctors ran tests, trying to determine the cause of the pain. At first they thought he might have a malignancy, but then, because of the low white blood count, they began to fear leukemia.

I almost died that week, sitting, waiting, walking the halls of Margaret R. Pardee Hospital in Hendersonville. Little did I realize how much time we were all going to spend there soon.

I sat so many days in that four-by-four waiting room that the walls began to close in on me. My spine seemed to be paralyzed. I stood, I walked the halls, I tried to read, but every time I did my eyelids threatened to close.

Suddenly, from nowhere, the doctor appeared. I started to get up. He smiled. "Don't get up," he said. "We can talk right here."

After a week of test tubes, X rays, and urinalyses, the doctor's diagnosis was a congenital kidney problem.

"Surgery is in order," he said. "We would like to schedule him for a nephroectomy."

"What is that?" I asked, fear mounting in my throat.

He hesitated. "That, Mrs. Shelton," he said, "is the removal of a kidney. In this case, the right kidney."

I was frightened almost out of my senses. Woody was numb. What a terrible thing to happen to a boy who had just turned seventeen!

We had to break the news to Danny. I felt this would be the hardest thing I would ever have to do.

Woody was unable to go into Danny's room. He was absolutely killed over the whole thing. He could never stand to see any hurt come to either of us, and he was really beside himself.

It would be up to the doctor and me to tell Danny. We went into his room. I was extremely nervous.

"Dan," the doctor said, "I have to tell you what is wrong with you. . . ." He dropped his head, groping for words. I turned to the window and stared at the buildings across the street, trying unsuccessfully to hold back the tears. The buildings blurred, and I felt tears trickling down my cheeks. They dropped on the windowseat. I stayed there so Danny could not see me cry.

Danny broke the silence. "What's wrong?" he asked. "I have a right to know." His voice was innocent and curious, his defenses down, his blue eyes wide open and staring straight at the doctor.

"Dan, you must have your right kidney removed," the doctor said.

As the doctor spoke, Danny studied his face, and finally, with a forced smile, he said, "I'm not worried, Mom. We can handle this."

I turned to him, and he saw the tears.

He smiled. "I'll be okay, Mom."

Once again, on October 6, 1968, I found myself sitting in that small waiting room across from the hospital pharmacy. Danny was in the operating room. I was alone. Woody had disappeared when Danny went to the operating room. He couldn't take it.

I have never figured out why those rooms are so small, or why someone can't be there to serve coffee or talk to members of the families who wait, and wait, and wait, under such trying circumstances. Outdated magazines lay all over the room, and the ashtrays overflowed. There was only one small window and far too much furniture.

I just couldn't stay put. I walked to the door and stood outside in the hall. I could see the large, heavy, swinging doors at the end of the hall that led to the operating rooms. On the right was intensive care; on the left were two large elevators to carry patients and visitors.

The hall was busy with nurses and other hospital personnel scurrying about. A worried husband stood at the corner, waiting for his wife to return from surgery. An exhausted lab technician passed by with a tray filled with blood samples.

After what seemed an eternity of watching the passing parade, the surgeon came through the double doors and hurried to me. He had a smile on his face.

"Dan is going to be fine," he said. "The surgery was successful. He'll be out of commission for a while, but don't worry—he will soon be back to normal."

"Thank you, Lord," I said, and began to cry. "And thank you, doctor."

The following weeks were intense and wearisome. After a month in the hospital, after intense pain and many shots, after much frustration and loss of weight, Danny was on his way to recovery.

He overcame victoriously. He returned to normal.

His life was to go on; God needed him here for a reason.

Dan later traveled for a year with a folk religious group, singing and witnessing. But that wasn't the reason God spared Dan; he had a more important task for him.

6

We were an average family with a modest income, but we made the most of it and lived comfortably. We owned a nice brick and wood home, complete with mortgage, three bedrooms, two baths, living room, family room, and garage. The patio out back was shaded by lovely oaks. Inside, the rooms were decorated in all our favorite colors.

Dan had completely recovered from the kidney operation. He did not return to the private school but finished high school in Hendersonville. As Dan grew on toward twenty, he and Woody continued to hunt and fish and enjoy the outdoors.

Ours was a normal, beautiful family life with no serious problems that we had not been able to handle. There was no immediate hint of Woody's impending illness. He continued to work at the paint store, and the change that came over him was so gradual that we could never pinpoint the start of it.

One day I realized that he had been acting strangely. He would leave the house without telling me, which had been alien to his nature for the twenty years we had been married. He would be gone the entire day and sometimes into the night. He showed irritation when I asked where he had been.

He became moody. He sat and stared into space, as if he were a thousand miles away.

He had always taken great pride in his cooking and was quite a good amateur chef, especially on warm summer evenings when he decided to cook outdoors on charcoal. The meals he prepared were delicious. But he tapered off his cooking and finally quit.

All sorts of thoughts ran through my head. Had he found another woman? Was our marriage going sour after twenty years, as many do? Surely this couldn't be happening to Woody and me!

Woody reached a point where he would not eat at the table with Dan and me. He came home from work in the afternoons and went straight to his room and closed the door. I could hear the commode flush, the shower run, and a few minutes later he would open his dresser drawers and closet doors; then there was silence and I knew he was dressing for bed.

That went on for a little more than two years. We became strangers in our own home.

Dan and I waited every day for him to come to dinner, but he would not. We ate in silence, and usually Dan would leave for the evening. When he heard Dan leave, Woody would get out of bed and walk down the hall to the kitchen. I always left his dinner on the table and in the oven. He would eat, never saying a word to me, never thanking me. When finished, he would silently return to his room and go back to bed. I wouldn't see him again until the next afternoon.

I lived in the guest room, and when Woody left for work each day I did not hear him. It was almost as if he slipped out secretly, as if he had something to hide. I wondered how much longer I could live like this without cracking up.

The first major explosion came in the fall of 1972,

around Dan's twenty-first birthday. Woody completely shut Dan out of his life, and he finally asked him to move out of our home.

Neither Dan nor I could understand what was happening. Dan had a job at the General Electric plant nearby. In March he rented a place at the Old Mill Apartments in Flat Rock and moved out of the house.

Soon after that, on his way home from work, Dan struck another car in the rear. He was not injured, but because of his previous kidney problem, any accident in which he was involved was a matter of concern. Woody, however, paid no attention to this accident. He did not even check to see if Dan had been hurt, or if he needed help. This was completely out of character for Woody, and I began to wonder exactly what was wrong with him.

I talked to our minister and tried to get Woody to talk to him, but he wanted no part of it. Then I begged Woody to see a doctor, and he refused, as I knew he would.

On Thanksgiving Day in 1972, I talked to Woody earnestly about going to the doctor, and he became so upset that he slapped me viciously, knocking me down the hallway. He had never struck me before. He stared at me lying on the floor, and a frown of wonderment crossed his eyes, but he just wheeled and walked out of the house.

He went to see my brother, Maurice, and told Maurice that he thought he was ill, that he was losing control of himself, but he didn't know why. Until then, he had maintained steadfastly that nothing was wrong with him. This was his first admission that he might be ill. He knew in the back of his mind that something was wrong, that he couldn't face things, but still he refused to see a doctor. He was fighting it in the only way he knew.

Early that spring, I became ill with severe chest pains, and the doctor admitted me to the hospital, suspecting a heart condition; but after extensive tests he discovered that I suffered from a type of globus syndrome caused by a good case of shot nerves. I had been living under growing strain for two years.

During the week I was in the hospital, Woody didn't bother to check by or even ask what was wrong. He did not come to visit me. Dan came every day, of course, and we didn't know how to take this from Woody. We didn't know whether he didn't want us and didn't care, or if he was really ill.

I had not told anyone except Woody and Dan that I was going to the hospital, not even my own family. Consequently no one came to visit me except Dan, the doctor once a day, and occasionally a nurse who took my temperature. I had plenty of time to think—and to feel sorry for myself.

A huge old oak tree stood outside my window, and I studied it for hours on end. It seemed to be telling me something. Late one afternoon, I took a pen and a piece of paper and began to write:

It is winter now, and as I sit by my window and view that old oak tree, I can see that he has been strong from many years of stress and strain. He must have had a heart attack, or a spastic colon, or, who knows? He may have just needed love as so many of us do—but he has weathered the storm well.

Most of his leaves are gone, but way down low, on the bottom branch, he has a few leaves still holding on, hoping and waiting for some love and sunshine.

When spring comes, I will view that same old oak,

and he will be standing tall and strong, recovered from what ailed him. He will have the love for which he waited so long.

I love that old oak tree!

As I read and reread the words I had written, I thought: Could that tree really be telling me something? Is he telling me that I can weather the storm? Or is he telling me to stop feeling sorry for myself, to get up off my rear and go solve my problem?

Whatever, I decided then and there that I was not going to give up. I would do what I thought best for Woody, Dan, and me—three people who were slowly suffocating.

I could not permit that to happen.

The day I was released from the hospital, Dan was working and Woody would not come to see me, so I called some friends and asked if they would be kind enough to come and take me home.

I had been feeling sorry for myself and expressed it quite openly, but my friends didn't want to hear about it. Around them, Woody was still the same old Woody, acting quite normally. It was only with Dan and me that he had changed so much. He had taken on a Jekyll-and-Hyde characteristic that, quite frankly, baffled me. It was so complex a puzzle that I couldn't begin to figure it out.

The ugly thought of separation coursed through my mind.

7

When my friends took me home from the hospital that day, I thanked them and went into the house alone. The house was cold and damp. Woody had been taking his meals out and using the house only for sleeping. Lately, he had lost interest in everything about our home.

As I walked through the house, tears streamed down my cheeks. I am an emotional woman.

The idea of separation was a last resort, but I had exhausted all other thoughts, and this one grew in my mind.

I would talk to Woody and try to convince him that we must work out some sort of arrangement for a separation on a trial basis. I could no longer stand the stifling life we had lived for two years, and I also had Dan to consider. I thought if Woody and I could be apart for a period of time, we might solve our problem. One thing was sure—we could not solve it living under the same roof. Apart, our minds might unclog.

We had been married twenty-two and one-half years. How time flies! I was grateful to Woody for those years. He had filled our lives with so many wonderful things. We had had valleys and peaks, but the good times, even considering the last two years, far outweighed the bad.

And the bad times had made us more appreciative of the good.

We did not have a lot materially, but we had been blessed in so many other ways. Still, I had to consider the things that had developed in the last two years.

Dan had moved out, but came by or called every day to see if we were all right. If Woody was at home when Dan came by, he would not talk to Dan. We suspected that Woody was ill, but we could not get him to see a doctor or try in any way to help himself and thereby help us.

I looked at myself. I used to think I was a whole person, but now I had become only half a woman, simply a framework of bone and flesh—no one inside, no one outside. Gradually, piece by piece, we were falling apart.

I can't let this happen, I thought. If I can't save Woody, then I must save Dan and myself.

I cleaned the house that afternoon, and as I entered each room I sat down for a moment, mentally going over the many years we had lived there.

It was a beautiful place to live. We had wonderful neighbors. Across the street a doctor and his wife had lived for many years, but both had recently died. Next to them were the Robinsons. Coy was a good friend to Woody. They were golfing partners. At the top of the circle lived the Holdens, who had three beautiful girls. To our left were Gerald and Ann Echols, who had moved into the neighborhood the summer past. They had two children, Beth and Danny. Danny was about seven, and we had especially enjoyed him. He was in and out of our house several times every day.

As I sat in the bedroom we had not shared for almost two years, I thought: I will give everything to Woody. Material things always had seemed to be so much more important to him than to me, despite the fact that he had lost interest in the house lately. Possibly that was because of my presence.

I made his bed the same as I had for more than twenty years. When I ran the vacuum under the bed, I found an old sock and a pair of brown bedroom slippers. I held them in my hand and thought of the Christmas I had given them to him, only a year or so ago. Now they were almost worn out.

One of the curtains on the window had gotten off its track. Before this, Woody never let anything remain broken or out of place. At times he almost drove me up the wall keeping the house clean and straight, but I quickly discovered this was better than someone who didn't care at all.

As I worked on the curtain, there was a knock at the back door. It was little Danny from down the street.

"Hi, Barbara," he said. "What'cha doing?"

"Hello, Danny," I said. "I'm cleaning the house. Come in."

We talked a couple of minutes. He fidgeted, looking around the house as if expecting someone.

Finally he said he had to go out to play. "I'll be back when Woody comes home," he said.

Woody had fun with little Danny. Since he couldn't be around our Dan, for whatever reason, he had found another Danny to take his place. This was really strange. He talked and laughed and played with Danny, and talked with another friend, Clay Richardson, a teenager, but would have nothing to do with Dan and me.

To other people, Woody was the same kind, gentle man he had been to us in the past, but he resented our presence, and his resentment had grown dramatically in recent weeks.

Dan and I often talked about this resentment, about how differently Woody treated us from others. We decided together that until we could work things out, it was best if we stayed away, letting his other friends help.

Clay and Danny were great for Woody, and this made Dan and me feel good, knowing that he had someone close that he could talk to, even if they were young.

I talked to Woody's family and our friends about his behavior, but I could tell they didn't believe what I told them because they only saw the one side of his character. They suspected, I could tell, that I just wanted to leave him, that I had grown tired of our marriage.

At this point, however, I felt that I couldn't waste time worrying about what people thought. I had to keep Woody, Dan, and myself from stifling.

Also, I could not blame others for not understanding. We didn't understand, either.

At 5:45 that afternoon, Woody came home. I felt that I must make the approach.

"Woody," I said, "can we sit down and talk?"

"No," he said. "I don't want to talk."

"We really need to," I said.

He stormed at me. "Just leave me alone," he screamed.

"Please, Woody," I tried to quiet him. "The neighbors will hear you."

"I don't care if the neighbors hear me," he shouted.

He rushed into his room and slammed the door.

I sat in silence for twenty minutes, and when I looked up, Woody was standing there. He was calm.

"What did you want to talk about?" he asked.

"Woody, we have to do something," I said. "We're falling apart. All three of us."

He didn't say anything.

"Can we separate on a trial basis?" I ventured.

He flared again. "No," he screamed. "I don't want any part of this."

"But, Woody. . . ."

"It's out of the question," he yelled. "Leave me alone. Get out of my life and leave me alone."

By this time we were both so angry there were no tears. I thought him to be completely irrational.

"I'll look for an apartment tomorrow," I said, and he must have sensed the finality in my voice. He went back in his room and stayed.

I was at that moment determined to make the break, or die trying. I telephoned Dan to tell him of my decision. I asked if he would like to share an apartment with me. On my salary, I probably couldn't afford the rent, especially in the approaching summertime, as Hendersonville is a resort town. Floridians pour into town in the spring and early summer, and rent values skyrocket. For that reason, Dan was eager to join me. The Old Mill Inn is a seasonal resort, and rent increases steeply in summer. Dan could no longer afford to live there.

As I searched for an apartment, a melancholy feeling came over me. I felt it would be impossible to move out of the house, but I had no choice. I hoped by leaving Woody that we could at least continue to be friends, even though we could not live as one. If I stayed with him longer, everything surely would be destroyed. By leaving, I thought we might be able to repair our lives.

I needed to continue to be friends with him, regardless of how far apart we grew. Children tie a man and wife together, and Dan was our bond.

In addition, I really wanted to help Woody, but there was a wall between us so high I couldn't climb it, so thick I couldn't break the barrier.

8

In early March of 1973, we found a small garage apartment on the edge of town. The location was a necessity since I had no transportation.

The apartment had one bedroom, a living room, one bath, and a tiny kitchen about the size of the bathroom. I had never realized that I would have to live in such cramped quarters again, and certainly I had no knowledge of the fact that my life would become much, much worse.

One bedroom was enough, since Dan worked all night at the plant, and I worked during the day with young people at the First Baptist Church. I slept at night, arose early each morning, and changed the bed linen for Dan, who slept during the day. Each night, I changed the linen back to mine. That was the most-changed bed in Henderson County! On weekends, Dan slept on the sofa in the living room, and I slept in the bed.

Until Woody changed, my life had been delightfully fragmented. I had been a dental assistant for fourteen years, and I had worked as a decorator. My job at the church gave me contact with people. But I could not shake the feeling that my first priority and primary joy in life was my role as wife and mother. In my present situation, I felt utterly bereft.

I believe strongly in the institution of marriage, and those who feel as I do know that a marriage must be worked with dedication. I had prayed that our marriage would hold up, and I had, indeed, worked at holding it together. So had Woody, until the last two years.

My feelings about marriage came partly from my deep religious faith, and partly from my upbringing. I grew up in the country, and that, I have always considered, was one of the greatest gifts my parents gave me.

Their marriage was idyllic, not because it was sweet and light, but because it was balanced and human. My father is small in size, but extremely large in strength. My mother is short, very quiet and generous, warm and wise in a gentle way, and always gives love. Neither ever squelches the other. They have experienced many personal and professional crises, but have never been defeated by them. In everything, their marriage came first.

From them I learned valuable lessons about marriage, about motherhood and devotion, about myself. I learned never to hurt anyone purposely, only to help and give love.

So why wouldn't Woody let us help him? I loved him very much. I would discover in a short while that I really hadn't known what true love is. The next two and one-half years would teach me the real meaning of our marriage vows. "Till death do us part" is a long time. How quickly we repeat the minister's words, and how soon we forget!

I felt a deep sorrow for Woody. He was alone. I had Dan, who had enriched, united, and challenged our relationship. He had brought to our lives immense happiness.

During the next four months, Dan and I looked for a

larger apartment. I got a job with an interior designer, and things began to look better. One day, a real estate woman told me of a vacant apartment across town. She said it was a lovely place upstairs in a private home. I telephoned the landlady and went straight over to see the apartment. Her name was Mary Sally, and we hit it off right away.

The apartment had two baths, two bedrooms, a living room, and a large kitchen. But it was unfurnished, and I had no furniture. Woody had it all. He had sold our home and bought a smaller one, and he still had the furniture.

Dan and I took the apartment anyway. The interior designer with whom I worked, Bill Smyth, was a fantastic artist. He drew plans for Dan and me, and I began to plan the decoration of the apartment. We ordered wallpaper, carpet, and paint, and began decorating, working days, nights, and weekends to get the apartment ready in a hurry.

On a Sunday afternoon that fall, my mother, father, and niece Melissa dropped by for the afternoon. I still had no furniture in the living room, and we all sat on the bed in the bedroom except Daddy, who sat in our only chair. I had hung curtains, and we were waiting for the carpet and other furnishings to arrive.

Mother had bad news. The three of them had stopped by to see Woody, and Mother was upset.

"Barbara," she said, "Woody wasn't able to hug Melissa's neck. He couldn't raise his right arm above his waist."

Tears came to our eyes. All my family loved Woody, and our separation had hurt the entire family. My mother was like a mother to Woody, and he worshipped her.

Dan had begun to visit Woody often, but said he had

noticed nothing strange about his physical abilities. After our separation, with me out of the picture, Woody had warmed up to Dan. He was quite friendly with him now, almost as if nothing had ever happened. Dan wanted to help him, and both Dan and I were happy that Woody had changed toward him. At that time, however, Dan was in photography school in Asheboro, North Carolina.

When my parents and Melissa left that afternoon, I tried to call Woody to ask what was wrong, but he didn't answer the phone. Once, as I tried to dial him, I looked out the window and saw his little car go by on the Asheville highway. I tried until late that night, but got no answer.

The next day, Monday, I knew he would be at work, so I telephoned him late in the afternoon when he got home. He answered immediately.

"Woody," I said, "what is wrong?"

"Nothing," he said. "There's nothing wrong. I don't have any problems, so don't worry about me."

"Listen, Woody," I said, "we're apart, but that doesn't mean that I don't love you. I want to know how you're feeling. Please tell me how your arm is bothering you."

He was silent.

"Woody, I'm very much concerned about you," I said. "Please tell me how you feel and what is wrong."

He finally said, "I'm not able to pick up a small pencil."

There was a silence between us; neither of us could say a word.

Instantly a fear came over me. I became as weak as water. The second he said he could not pick up a pencil, I knew something was terribly wrong with him.

I could hear him sobbing quietly on the other end of the line.

When I regained my composure, I said, "Woody, you

are an intelligent man. You thought arthritis was your problem, but you must know by now that it isn't your only problem."

I could hear him sniffling, and I envisioned tears flowing down his cheeks. The thought came to me that now was the time we could get back together and perhaps repair our marriage.

"If I can get you an appointment," I asked, "will you go to the doctor? Please, Woody."

Apparently he had finally faced the fact that something was seriously wrong, and he seemed to want help. He did not discourage me, or ask me to hang up. He said he would see the doctor.

"Woody," I plunged farther, "is there a possibility that I can see you?"

"Yes," he said, "but not now. Wait till I see the doctor."

I was encouraged with the hope of reconciliation, and early the next morning I telephoned the office of Dr. Chris McConnachie, an orthopedic surgeon in Hendersonville, and made an appointment for Woody.

Dr. McConnachie examined Woody in late September 1973. He found Woody's illness to be in the horn cells family, but he said it was out of his field and referred Woody to Drs. Sellers and Lampley.

They confirmed the diagnosis of amyotrophic lateral sclerosis and sent Woody to Winston-Salem for an appointment with Dr. E. H. Martinot in the orthopedic surgery and rehabilitation center of Bowman Gray Hospital. Dr. Martinot did electromyographs and nerve conduction studies of Woody's arms and legs, confirmed the diagnosis of ALS again, and repeated what Woody had been told by Drs. Sellers and Lampley—terminal illness with no known cure.

I waited for Woody to call and tell me the results of

the examinations, but he didn't call. I was so anxious that I went to see Drs. Sellers and Lampley, and they told me the truth. They told me the extent of the illness, and what the result would be—death. They also said they wanted Woody to visit Dr. Cecil T. Durham, Jr., an Asheville neurosurgeon, for yet another opinion.

This was crushing news. I went home immediately and telephoned Woody.

"Can I come to see you now?" I asked.

"Yes," he said simply.

I left the apartment immediately and drove the three blocks to his house. Strange, I thought, how two people could live three blocks apart in a small town and see each other only twice in six months. He had constantly avoided me, fighting a battle within himself.

When I reached Woody's house, I could not believe my eyes. He had bought a home on the side of a hill, with a long flight of steps leading to the door. He had not known that in a short while he would be unable to walk them. As I slowly walked up the steps, I counted them—one, two, three—wondering what I would say when I got inside—four, five, six. What would I do? How would I feel?

I didn't think Woody knew what his illness really was. Should I tell him? Should I wait and tell him later?

How will he receive me? Will he take me in his arms and hold me close, or will he treat me like a stranger?

All these questions raced through my head, and when I reached the porch I was lightheaded and breathless. I rang the bell, and the door slowly opened.

Woody was as handsome as ever, but his face was sad and drawn as if he had been crying. He didn't say, "Come in," he simply stepped back. I didn't know whether to hug him, shake his hand, or just walk in. He made no effort to touch me, so I walked in. He indicated a chair and asked me to sit down.

The house was small but very clean. I knew it would be clean, for he was an immaculate person. It had two bedrooms, one bath, a living room and kitchen, and a small sunroom at one side. Beside the sunroom was a patio.

He had a lot of flowers, but they hadn't been watered and were dying. That, in itself, tipped off his condition, for he had a green thumb and would never let anything die if he could help it.

We talked animatedly, and I got the feeling that he wanted me to help, but couldn't find the words to ask. I told him that if he wanted help, all he had to do was call. I assured him that both Dan and I wanted to help him, but he was such an independent, self-sufficient person that it had to be his choice for me to come back.

I had brought a basket of chicken for his dinner, and as he ate he said, "I'll think about your coming back to care for me, and let you know if you can."

"Dan and I are the only ones who really understand," I said. "We would care for you completely."

"I know," he said. "You both are great!"

His words thrilled me. At last, I thought, we're about to work out a reconciliation.

I got up, kissed him on the top of his head, and left for my apartment to await his call.

I had visited him on Wednesday evening. I slept very little that night, thinking about his illness. All day Thursday I waited by the phone, but he did not call.

Friday morning, I was taking a bath when the phone rang. I leaped from the tub, grabbed a towel, and ran to answer the phone.

"Barbara," Woody said, "did you mean what you said about coming back and taking care of me?"

"Yes," I breathed.

"I'd like you and Dan to come for dinner tonight," he said. "I'll fix steaks."

That was as near as he could bring himself to say "yes"—and it was enough for me. "We'll be there around six," I said.

Dan came home from school in Asheboro about four that afternoon, planning to go to a high-school football game. I was in Dr. Lampley's office at the time, trying to learn more about Woody's illness.

I dreaded telling Dan about his father's illness, and I knew I couldn't tell him over the phone. I called him, though, to tell him to wait for me at the apartment, that I had something to tell him. He knew from the tone of my voice that something was seriously wrong.

"Mom," he asked, "what's the matter?"

"I can't tell you over the phone," I said. "Just wait for me, please."

There was silence on the phone. I knew he was disturbed. He always knew when something was wrong.

"Okay, Mom," he said. "I'll be here when you get home."

I left the doctor's office and quickly drove home. Dan was in his room, sitting on the bed. I sat on the other side of the bed and told him about his father, of the illness, and how tragic it was. I told him the doctors said Woody was going to die no matter what we did, and that we could go back to care for him.

"Dan," I said, "he invited us to dinner tonight."

We looked at each other then in silence, and we each began to cry. He took my hand in his and held it tightly.

"You know, Mom," he said, "God promised that he would never leave us, never give us more than we can stand. We must believe."

Woody and I had always thought of Dan as "our little boy," but at that moment he was as much of a man as I ever knew.

Suddenly, the wallpaper, the paint, the carpet samples,

and the few pieces of furniture scattered around were not as important as they had been. The only thing that mattered was our keen awareness that our Lord was always near. Nothing like his presence can dispel the fear and terror of the unknown.

Thoughts ran through our heads: We live uncertain lives; only God knows what the future will bring. Any hour could bring disaster—Woody could die at any moment. We would have to live one day at a time.

9

At 6 o'clock we drove to Woody's little house on the hill. Neither of us spoke. I'm sure Dan's mind was working overtime; mine surely was.

The dinner went smoothly. Woody dropped the steaks several times, not having the strength to hold them, but we pretended not to notice.

He wanted to prepare dinner himself, without any help, and through pure stubbornness he did. He made a tossed green salad, baked potatoes, and set out sour cream and butter. In the oven he had rolls and blackberry pie.

Dan placed the plates on the patio table, and I found an old candle someone had given Woody and put it in the center.

We made senseless conversation, talking about the weather, the house, everything but the actual problem. When the steaks were ready, Dan carried them to the table. Woody, walking to his place at the table, tripped and stumbled. He almost fell. "That's crazy," he laughed. "I stumble all the time. I don't know why."

Dan and I glanced at each other. Woody didn't realize how tragically ill he was. Even we did not know how far his illness had progressed.

We tried to keep cheerful at the table, but it was impossible. This was the first time we three had eaten together in two years, and our emotions were running high.

The food lodged in my throat and wouldn't go down. Dan nibbled at his steak as if he had a week to eat it. Woody had trouble trying to cut his steak. Dan reached over and began to cut his father's steak, and Woody began to cry.

"Don't cry, Dad," Dan said. "Everything will be all right."

Smoke from the charcoal fire blew across the table and gave Dan and me an excuse to wipe tears from our eyes without Woody's suspecting that we were crying. The pungent odor of the charcoal reminded me of the many pleasant evenings we had spent at Lake Lure.

Woody and I did the dishes, and Dan went on to the football game. "Mom," he said as he left, "call me if you need me."

Woody and I moved into the living room. I lay down on the sofa, and Woody sat in a big, brown armchair with his feet propped on the footrest.

For a long while, we didn't talk. I stared around the room. It was decorated in browns and beiges, but pleasing and comfortable. It looked like a man's place.

The fireplace at the backside of the room had been painted the same color as the walls, antique white, a special formula that Woody had mixed for our house. I looked at the ceiling and thought how strange that Woody had used the very same colors that I had used in our previous home.

A large mirror, a fraction off-center, hung over the fireplace, and two brass lamps rested on heavy, maple end tables on each side of the brown and yellow floral sofa. Fresh cigarette butts were snubbed in an ashtray on

one end table, and I thought Woody must have had company that afternoon. He didn't smoke.

At one end of the room was a large painting of a colos-
sal black bear standing at the trunk of a huge tree with a
hole in its base. That was Woody's type of painting.

I wondered what thoughts he was thinking. He had
given no indication that he had knowledge of his illness,
and somehow I had to explain it to him.

"Woody," I asked, "have the doctors told you what's
wrong?"

"Yes," he said slowly. "But I shut it out. I didn't listen."

"Why not?"

"Because it's bad," he said, "and I don't want to
know."

From bits of the previous conversation, I was sure that
Woody thought he had cancer. The doctors had attempted to explain to him that he suffered from
amyotrophic lateral sclerosis, but he had shut it completely out of his mind.

As we talked, he kept his eyes closed.

"Woody, open your eyes," I said. "I'm going to tell
you what's wrong with you."

He opened his eyes wide and appeared to be looking
right through me.

"Do you remember Lou Gehrig?" I asked.

He nodded.

"You must remember the illness he had."

He nodded again.

"That's what's wrong with you, Woody," I said. "It is
a rare illness." I phrased my words carefully, but said
them plainly. "There is no known cure. The doctors say
there is a possibility you will lose the use of your right
arm, and your left arm, and possibly your legs."

The only thing I didn't tell him was that he would also

lose his speech. Telling him all of it might have been too much of a shock to his nerves.

"Dan and I will be with you as long as you need us and want us," I added. "Don't you ever forget that."

For several minutes he sat silently, then he struggled out of the chair and began watering his flowers. He went to the kitchen and scooped a bowl of ice cream for me. He set the bowl on an end table and sat down on the sofa next to me. He took me in his arms and held me closely, and we both began to weep.

"Woody, we'll fight this together," I said, "the three of us."

"Yes," he said, "we're going to make it."

He began to soften, as if a thousand pounds had been taken off his shoulders. He did not know how ill he actually was, or how helpless he would become. He was relieved to learn he did not have cancer; he had a great fear of cancer and associated it with sure death. He did not realize that what he had was worse, an illness that cannot be cured or even checked.

In times of trouble and fear, most of us are unable to cope with the cruel circumstances and unanswered complexities of life. Often our first impulse is to run away and hide.

Woody had done that, but now he was out of hiding.

My husband and I got on our knees before the sofa and prayed: "Lord, we give ourselves to you because we can't take care of ourselves. We have been apart. Forgive us. And show us your will."

Silently, we renewed our marriage vows.

When we arose, I felt a contentment engulf me, and Woody appeared to be at peace.

I was overjoyed: Dan and I were coming home.

10

In the midst of our misfortune and near-panic, an awareness slowly seeped into us that we were not alone. We felt God's great hand on our shoulders. His presence threw a different light on our problem. Suddenly, things were not as dark as they had been.

We gave ourselves to him completely, and he in turn gave us the strength to cope—a strength that was unbelievable.

Those who experience a tragic and challenging illness such as ALS usually do one of two things: They begin to feel sorry for themselves and become bitter, or they accept their fate and try to enrich themselves through it.

We felt we couldn't leave everything to God. Given his strength, we were willing to do the work. We were his instruments, Dan and I, and when Dan returned to school in early October, I left the apartment and moved into the house with Woody. My parents, happy over our reconciliation, but knowing we were in for a long siege, moved back to Hendersonville from Woodruff to be near us and to help in any way they could. In the months to come, they would be towers of strength.

Woody and I visited Dr. Durham, the neurologist in Asheville, who reiterated that there was no known cure. Dr. Durham told us that a cobra serum, administered directly from the snake, had been used in ALS victims, but to date there were no successful results on record.

"The only encouragement I can give you," Dr. Durham said, "is that in certain cases the cobra serum has prolonged life."

"No," Woody said. "I don't want it. If I get to the point that I can't move, I don't want to live in that condition."

At last, Woody was being realistic. Apparently he had accepted the fact that, barring a miracle, he was going to die regardless of what we did.

I still wondered about Woody's strange behavior the last two and one-half years, and asked Dr. Durham, "Does this illness affect a person psychologically?"

"Why do you ask?" he asked.

"For more than two years," I said, "Woody has been a different man. His personality changed." I explained Woody's actions toward Dan and me.

"I see," Dr. Durham mused. "Yes," he said, "we don't know why, but most ALS patients go through a period of great psychological stress. Quite often they do things they don't remember doing."

I asked Dr. Durham every question I could think of about the illness we faced. I wanted to learn as much as possible. I believe understanding a problem is a great step toward solving it, or, in our case, toward coping with it.

We returned to Hendersonville in the certainty that Woody's fate was sealed. Each of the doctors we had visited were kind and understanding. They had given us all the information available, and they were more than willing to help, but their hands were tied. They could offer diagnosis and advice, but very little help.

Dr. Sellers and Dr. Lampley stood with us through it all, and we followed their advice closely in caring for Woody.

"Give Woody his way," Dr. Sellers advised. "He will be frustrated enough, and the less you allow him to be upset, the better he will feel."

We lost some friends because of this, friends who did not understand, who meant well, but who could not resist talking of things that upset Woody.

I would have climbed the highest mountain to keep from upsetting him, and Woody quickly came to the realization that he was easily frustrated. "Don't let anyone upset me," he said almost every day. "I can't handle it. My nerves are shot. Whatever you do, Barbara, protect me from that."

I never told him anything I thought might disturb him. He worried constantly about finances, and the only deceitful thing I did was to keep two checkbooks—one with our correct balance in it, which I used, and the other with an inflated balance to show him. That way, he thought we had money when we didn't, and he did not worry.

I leveled with him about everything else. This honesty helped him considerably. He knew when he asked a question of me that he would get a straight answer.

I was grateful that he never asked about dying. I'm not sure I could have handled that.

Dr. Lampley warned that many ALS victims die of heart attacks, and we determined to avoid that, if possible. That was one reason we tried to protect Woody from disturbance.

"Secretion," Dr. Lampley said, "should never be allowed to accumulate in Woody's lungs. That would increase the danger of pneumonia." So we constantly moved him, and when he became helpless and bedridden we constantly turned him.

"He could die from choking," Dr. Lampley said.

How horrible and frightening to choke to death! We lived in fear of that, and watched Woody closely, day and night, especially when he ate.

I wanted to learn more, and I didn't want to take up the time of busy physicians unnecessarily, so I went to the Hendersonville Public Library. The only information I found there was that ALS was an illness in the horn cells family that worked from the lateral part of the spine, deteriorating all voluntary muscles.

I checked out a book on the life of Lou Gehrig and read it, hoping it would give me hints on caring for Woody, but it was mostly the story of his baseball career, and I found nothing of great use in it. However, it was an extremely inspiring story of a great athlete and a great man.

I telephoned the Multiple Sclerosis Foundation in Charlotte and asked for any literature on ALS. In a few days, I received a pamphlet in the mail which contained almost word for word the information that Dr. Lampley and Dr. Sellers had already given me.

"The usual form of the disease is widespread, and gradual loss of strength and muscle control due to damage centers in the brain and spinal cord," the pamphlet read. "The symptoms first appear in later life and are seen mostly through ages 40 to 70 years, with most cases rarely appearing before or after these ages. It is more common in men than in women, and is found in all races and countries. It has been estimated that between five and ten thousand cases exist in the United States at any given time. This makes the illness extremely rare. The life span is from one to three years, and five at the most. . . ."

There are about twenty different varieties of muscle control diseases. ALS is the most severe and most rapid of all. The symptoms vary and depend on the control centers involved in the damaging process. Motor nerve damage results in wasting and weakness of the muscles.

Early symptoms are irregular spasmodic twitching in small muscle fiber groups. This is called "fibrillation."

The twitching first appeared in Woody's right arm, and stayed until the arm was completely lifeless. Once he lost the strength in the arm, the twitching disappeared.

He then began to have the same twitching in his left arm, as though the muscles were fighting to survive.

He experienced a lot of burning, itching, and discomfort with the fibrillation. But all of it disappeared when each part of his body died.

Because of the burning and itching, he had to have many baths every day. I showered him twice each day, and gave him sponge baths when he became uncomfortable. They seemed to ease him.

What do you do to help a person you love, a person you know will become so fixed in his body that his mind will become a prisoner? It was up to Dan and me to work as closely with Woody as we possibly could, doing anything we could to make his life more comfortable. For many years, he had done that for us.

We never said "no" to a dying man.

11

The power of a positive mental attitude has always amazed me. When I began thinking of ways we could help Woody, of things we could do for him, I began talking to him a little each day about this principle. I had to work slowly with him. He did not share my feelings on positive thinking.

Gradually, by talking a little each day about how we were going to cope with his illness, and about how we would not think any farther than today, we were able to overcome many obstacles. Attitude became a prime importance in treating him.

I continued my own learning process. How, I thought one day, does it feel to be unable to move?

I sat perfectly still for a minute or two. It was difficult to sit that long without moving. In succeeding weeks, once or twice each day, when I came upon a quiet period, I sat very still, gradually lengthening the time I sat without moving, trying to accomplish within my own body the feeling Woody would experience when he reached the point where he couldn't move. To this day, I can sit for twenty or twenty-five minutes without moving anything but my eyes.

Woody was the ill one, but God had given me the talent and understanding to care for him, and I walked many miles in his moccasins. From those experiences, I learned.

We lay on the patio one day, Woody and I, luxuriating in the warm sunshine. Woody reclined in his swimsuit on the redwood chaise lounge, and I stretched out on my back on a blanket, gazing at the clouds floating across the sky.

A gorgeous redbird nibbled his lunch from the feeder at the top of the steps. He alternately pecked at the food and stared at us, as if he feared we would shoo him away.

"How beautiful and free he is," Woody said. We had every sort of bird you could imagine feeding in our garden that summer. They became so friendly and relaxed that they lost almost all fear of us.

"Woody," I asked, "do you remember when the illness began?"

He thought a few moments.

"No," he said. "It's like your foot going to sleep. You don't realize it until it's happened."

He pondered the question a few more minutes.

"It's strange," he said. "I think I've had it for a long time. My right arm has been bothering me for several years."

"Do you remember when you went to the doctor a few years ago and got those cortisone injections in your right elbow?" I asked. "Your arm ached so that you were unable to work for two or three weeks. I wonder if you could have had the illness then?"

"I don't know," he said, shaking his head.

Aware of the predicted life-span of three to five years, I suppose I was trying to pinpoint the beginning to get some idea of the impending end.

Woody had always appeared to be in near-perfect physical condition, though occasionally he became clumsy. If anything was ever turned over at the table, I knew Woody was responsible. He had constantly dropped things the last few years, and when we were at the lake he often fell in the water. Could the disease have been building within him for several years?

On a cold December day several years ago, Woody and a friend, Bill Brown, were working on the boathouse at Lake Lure when Woody fell in the icy lake.

Bill's wife, Charlotte, and I had cooked dinner and were driving it down to the lake when Woody suddenly whizzed by us like a streak, going back up the mountain.

We wondered where he was going, and when we got to the lake Bill was still laughing as he told us Woody had gone home for dry clothing. We kidded him for years about falling in the lake in December. Now, looking back, I'm not so sure he could have helped falling.

As I recall some of the times he fell or experienced clumsiness, it seemed as if he momentarily lost his strength.

"Could you have been affected that far back?" I asked. "Do you remember if you momentarily lost your strength?"

"I can't remember," he said, "but there must have been something wrong even then. I suppose we'll never know for sure."

We decided that since the doctors knew little about ALS, we would make notes and tapes, recording Woody's physical decline, and perhaps even film him during the illness. We hoped by doing this that we could help others cope with the fearful disease.

Woody was eager to help, but as the illness progressed, each time Dan took out the camera to photograph him, Woody would commence to cry. We decided that photographing him was out of the question, that it would be cruel and punishing to burden him with that. Although we were unable to take pictures, we talked often of the effects of the illness, and I kept notes and tapes.

Woody's life took on a different meaning. He began to change. Before this, he was a quiet person. He seldom talked much, and never shared his thoughts with us. Now he wanted to talk—needed to—and he talked constantly, telling us everything.

We passed a lot of time watching the birds playing around our patio. Woody sat out there for hours admiring them. Margie and Harold O'Dell came often to visit. They knew how much Woody loved the birds, and one day brought him a book on birds. We studied the book and soon could identify the different species. We named them and noticed that the same birds returned every day. We marveled at the pleasure they gave us.

Margie and Harold were a source of strength to us. In 1968 they lost their fourteen-year-old son to a brain tumor. The tumor was discovered when Hal was two and one-half, and they lived twelve years with the knowledge that he would never grow up.

When he was eleven, the doctors were forced to operate to insert a shunt into his jugular vein to relieve pressure on his brain. The operation cost him his sight, but he was a brave young man. He learned to read and play many games in braille.

His grandmother gave him a braille watch for Christmas, and he laughed and hugged my neck when he came to the dentist for his appointment. He showed me the watch, made me close my eyes and try to tell the time, and laughed when I couldn't.

I wanted to hold him in my arms and tell him that he would be well, but I knew this could never be.

During the years of Hal's illness, Margie and Harold displayed a courage that was beyond comprehension. God gave them fantastic strength to bear such a cross. Each day they watched little Hal's frail body gradually deteriorate, and they were unable to alter his tragic fate.

Margie and Harold had much compassion and understanding for Woody. God gave them a strength to overcome their sorrow and to comfort their young son, and now, five years after Hal's death, they shared that strength with us.

Grief can take care of itself, but to receive the full value of joy you must have someone to divide it with. The O'Dells taught us that.

Woody and I talked hours and hours, sharing, giving, trying to cram everything we could into every day. We tried not to lose a single minute.

We began to explore thoughts we'd never dreamed of discussing.

It is astonishing how we go through life every day, doing our chores, noticing little, and when we are suddenly faced with death, life becomes a revelation. The whole world becomes a beautiful heaven, a place we don't want to leave.

I believe God meant for us to have heaven on earth in the first place, and we made it a hell.

As I walked with Woody that summer, I walked with a friend. I wished each day would never end. I was so glad that he was there to help me realize how beautiful my world really is. I had faced the fact that Woody was dying, but suddenly I found myself crying out, "Not now! Please, not now! Let him live a little longer. Let us do a few more things together."

If he could live long enough, there was the possibility of discovery of a miracle drug—always the hope for a cure. But we knew deep down that this was false hope.

Somehow, we kept it in the backs of our minds, never wanting to let go. Doctors had told me there had been a number of cases in which ALS had arrested itself. They didn't know why, but this was also a hope.

We clung to hope—any hope.

12

The 1973 holidays approached, and we decided to spend Thanksgiving as usual with my family in Woodruff, South Carolina. Woody looked forward to the occasion and made the eighty-mile trip in good shape.

So many relatives gathered in my parents' home that it was impossible to convene around the table. People with plates sat all over the patio, in the den, and on the lawn. We gave thanks that we were all still together.

No one talked about Woody's condition, though it was known to all. They pushed it out of their minds and thought only of the terrific times we had when we all got together.

The nieces and nephews were there, and Woody had a way with children that was extraordinary. They loved him, and the knowledge of his illness and impending death was intense in their minds. Woody joined them for a game of kickball. The November sun was warm, and some of the kids wore shorts. Woody laughed when he kicked at the ball and missed. He couldn't find the co-ordination to connect his foot with the ball. The children laughed, too, but in the backs of their minds they wondered if this would be their last game with Uncle Woody.

The day passed rapidly, and when the time came for

departure, our hearts were heavy. Woody looked at everyone in a way that made our hearts ache, and he began to cry. Everyone joined him, and tears flowed.

One by one, my relatives hugged him, and we left. We drove the eighty miles home in near silence. Our guardian angel rode with us, for I don't remember any of that trip.

The mountains of North Carolina that fall had been like a fairyland, and now the golden leaves had turned to brown and fell from the trees. Woody mentioned the loveliness of it all, sometimes with cloudy eyes.

Many times that late autumn and early winter, we drove in the mountains for hours, talking occasionally, but mostly enjoying a silent companionship and marvelling at the handiwork of God.

Deep in our minds, however, were sobering thoughts: Woody was going to die. When? Would this be our last drive? How much longer?

The holidays were the hardest time we had experienced yet. Christmas was a beautiful time each year, our favorite holiday, and I suppose that's why it was so hard this year. The music was lovely, the stores were gaily decorated, and the church pageants were beautiful. We had known the extent of Woody's illness for two months. Despite the beauty around us, it was hard to get into the Christmas spirit.

Woody's progress in the three weeks leading to Christmas was good. In some ways he was his old self, almost the same as before illness struck him. He remained interested, inquisitive, and talked about everything. He was concerned with why so much had happened to him. When he put the question to me, I could only say that I didn't know, that God alone knew the answer. I often wondered why a man as good as Woody had to face such a tragic thing.

From great pain and suffering can come great richness, if you put your trust in God. Woody's spiritual life grew during those Christmas days. He read constantly, hungrily, from a large-print Bible that his brother Chester gave him when he became ill. He continued to read that Bible until he couldn't read any more.

He loved the twenty-third Psalm, and we read and reread the Christmas story. I don't know that Woody had ever read all of it.

We talked often about God and about Woody's relationship with God. Woody had rededicated his life to Christ, and when he did he went forward and was baptized. He wanted to be in church every time a service was scheduled, and on communion day he especially wanted to go, whether he felt like going or not. He wanted to partake of the body of Christ.

After his rededication, Woody became quite open in his discussion of God, something he had never been able to do before.

As we read the Bible together, certain passages came to hold great meaning for me. I drew great strength from a passage in the one hundred-sixteenth Psalm: "For thou hast delivered my soul from death, mine eyes from tears, and my feet from falling. I will walk before the Lord in the land of the living."

We knew that Woody would die, and that I would continue to live. That passage told me that my life must have meaning.

Perhaps the most meaningful Scripture, however, was Matthew 25:34–36, 40: "Then shall the King say unto them on his right hand, Come, ye blessed of my Father, inherit the kingdom prepared for you from the foundation of the world: For I was an hungered, and ye gave me meat: I was thirsty, and ye gave me drink: I was a stranger, and ye took me in: Naked, and ye clothed me: I was sick, and ye visited me; I was in prison, and ye came unto me . . . . Verily I say unto you, Inasmuch as ye have done it unto one of the least of these my brethren, ye have done it unto me."

I gave Woody all my time because he could not care for himself. I followed God's instructions in caring for him, even at the expense of giving time to my friends.

I believe that every person comes into our lives for a purpose—either to give or to receive—and if I don't take the time to respond to their needs, then I am not following God's plan for me.

Yes, I grew in as many ways that Christmas as did Woody.

He thought of his family, and occasionally I would see him crying. When I asked what was wrong, he would say that he loved his family and would like to see them. He said he wished he lived closer to them so he could see his brothers and sisters more often.

He needed constant reassurance that everyone cared for him. Years before, he didn't need me to tell him that I loved him. He knew I did. Now it became important for him to hear the words, "I love you." He wanted to be sure. As his illness progressed, he needed more and more love.

"Barbara," he said one day, "whatever you do, don't stop loving me."

The snow was beautiful that winter, but the weather was moderate. We thanked God for this. The cold brought torturing chills to Woody's body, due mostly, I'm sure, to his poor circulation. The extremely cold days, what few we had, were hard on him.

Though Woody could still walk, and on most days drive the car, each day brought new pains and different feelings within him. We worked hard to keep him comfortable and content, but the things that worked one day might not work the next. It became almost like working with a different person each day. His condition was so strange that we always had to work with him with an open mind.

He continued to work at the paint store with his old friend, Buddy Richardson. There were many days that he didn't feel like going to work, but he pushed on. He was unable to hold a pencil. The only way he managed to write was for me to wrap the end of a pencil with tape. He could pick up the pencil with his left hand, place it in his right hand, and with his left hand press his right fingers tightly to the tape. Then he could scribble.

He constantly dropped his pencil, cans of paint, and papers in the store. But his mind was sharp. People asked him what was wrong, and when he tried to tell them, he broke down and wept. He upset some of the customers, who shied away from him, and some of them upset him. He came home several times from work and said, "People just don't understand. They say things they don't mean." But he would never repeat what they had said.

It is hard, he knew, to talk to a dying man.

Before long, everyone in town who knew Woody knew of his illness. Our phone began to ring, and friends wanted to know if they could help. They let us know that they cared in many different ways, and this meant so much. Cards, letters, and calls poured in from everywhere.

"My friends tell me not to worry," Woody said one afternoon when he came in from work. "They slap me on the back and say, 'Don't worry. Everything will be all right.' But, Barbara, how can I keep from worrying? It's easy for them to say don't worry when they are so healthy."

13

By March 1974, Woody had lost the use of his right arm and had much trouble walking. Sometimes he used a cane, holding it in his left hand. He fell often. He was like a tree cut off at the base of the trunk. When he fell, he gave no warning, yet he never got hurt. The disease had so relaxed his muscles that he was sometimes like an inebriated man. He did not have the strength to catch himself.

He could no longer get up from a chair, so we made him a higher chair, which helped some. Even though he could not get up by himself, he felt a constant need to move. He could not sit still, and quite often I helped him up fifteen times or more a day.

I devised a way of lifting him, placing my knee against his knee and my arms on each side of his shoulders. With a backward movement, I was able to lift him with greater ease. I developed muscles you wouldn't believe.

The story of the man lifting the calf came to my mind and made me chuckle. It was said that if a man lifted a calf every day from the day it was born, he should be able to lift it when it became a cow.

By working with Woody gradually, lifting him every day, I could soon lift his 175 pounds. Woody had gained some weight in his forties. I only weighed 124, but I found that by doing things gradually I could surprise even myself.

By the end of March, Woody could no longer work. I had to dress him each day and give him showers. He couldn't tie his shoes, button his shirts, or zip his trousers.

We had little income after both our salaries terminated. When Woody could no longer work, I had to quit my job to stay home and care for him. We learned a different lifestyle in the next few months, but this did not trouble me. All my life I had taught myself to improvise. God had prepared me for this day for a long time. He had taught me to take nothing and make something beautiful out of it.

We knew that Woody's illness would be expensive, but I never had any doubts that we would be able to pay the bills. We had insurance, and we drew Social Security checks to supply our immediate household needs.

There were a number of relatives and friends who helped us financially. God worked through them. We had many people who prayed for us in the churches and homes, and we felt the effects of those prayers. My trust in God was also a trust in my fellowman.

Never did I get on my knees and say, "God, send us the money to pay these bills." At low moments in our lives someone always knocked on the door and came in to fill our void. Just at the point when we would get down to nothing financially, someone would call and say, "Barbara, we had a little money left over this month and I'm sending it to you." Or I would simply walk to the mailbox one day and help would be there in a letter.

We drew two hundred dollars a month from the Veterans Administration during that first year of Woody's illness, but when we filled out eligibility forms at the end of the year, we discovered that the severance pay

Woody received was above allowable limits, so we had to repay the government the money they had given us. The checks we would have received the second year were kept by the VA as repayment.

God performed many miracles during Woody's illness. He gave me understanding and the ability to care for Woody. We never came to a crossroad we couldn't cross. Sometimes we had to pause, but not for long. Through faith, we managed to break many barriers.

I thought many times of what Dan said when he learned the seriousness of his father's illness: We had to believe and to trust. God had promised never to give us more than we could stand.

The key word, I thought, was "trust." The word means that you give yourself to someone and completely believe that he will take care of you. I relate to the positive. I had complete trust in God; I have always had that trust. I knew that as long as we didn't lose sight of the meaning of this key word, we were all right. Woody was entrusted to our care, and we conditioned our minds and bodies to this kind of thinking.

I talked to other women who had battled terminal illness in their husbands. They said they were driven to the point of exhaustion long before the illness terminated. Many times I wondered if Woody's illness would destroy Dan and me before it took Woody's life, and those were the times when my faith slipped a little. But I had to renew it and live one day at a time.

14

March departed quietly, and April and May were beautiful months. We were able to get out more. The sky spread huge, billowy, low-hanging clouds across our town. The air was light and soft and fresh. Beautiful blossoms on the trees brought forth a fragrance that permeated the air. The shrubs turned green, and millions of flowers burst into bloom.

The fourth of June was Woody's forty-eighth birthday. I wondered if he were looking back across the years. We sat on the patio that day, and I thought of so many things that had happened to him in those forty-eight years. I had been in his life for almost half of them, but even then he had been partly alone. He never shared his thoughts with me unless I pulled them from him. He seldom discussed things with me, but seemed to think that I should know without having to hear it. If I had to question him, he felt I was prying, so to keep friction at a minimum, I learned to read between the lines, to ascertain without asking. I concentrated on interpreting his thoughts by his actions, little realizing through all those years that this would help me overcome the barrier of Woody's inability to speak, which would come soon.

Looking back, Woody's lack of communication through the years still bothered me. What had made him like that? Why had he been so alone? Was it me? Had I turned him off all those years?

I would never have the answers to those questions. All I knew was that after many years of marriage, he suddenly needed to be close, intimately close. We were now closer than ever; a bond held us tightly together, one that we had not possessed before.

I was glad that Woody felt the need to talk, to share himself with me at last. All those years, I had felt shut out, but now I had become an integral part of Woody's life—I felt whole.

Easter was early that year, but lovely as always. As I dressed Woody that morning, he placed his arms around my waist and kissed me on the forehead. He was only strong enough to raise his arms to my waist, and when he pressed I could barely feel a slight squeeze. In his mind, he felt as if he were holding me tight, but his body was unable to respond. The limpness of his body brought a chill to me, and when I turned away so that he couldn't see, I felt tears roll down my cheeks and drop onto the carpet.

I dressed him in a navy blue suit with white shirt and dark tie. I had to button the shirt, knot the tie, zip his trousers, and tie his shoes.

Woody came from a religious family, but had never attended church much in his adult life. The advent of his illness had brought to him a new-found and very deep faith, and he wanted to go to church whenever he was able.

We walked to the car, and I asked him to let me drive. He said, "No, as long as I'm able, I'm going to drive." He could handle nothing as small as the key, but he had attached a long bolt to it and could turn that. He had no use of his right arm, but still had strength to drive with his left. I worried about his driving, about his reflexes if he had to stop quickly, but I could not talk him out of it.

As we drove to the little Methodist Church in the country—the Tracy Grove Wesleyan Methodist—we passed a new cemetery on a hill. Woody remarked how beautiful the flowers were.

"This would be a nice place to be buried," he said, and turned the car into the cemetery.

"Please, Woody, don't stop here," I said. "We'll be late for church." I thought if he started talking about dying, I would not make it through the service.

He paid no attention to me.

"Barbara," he asked, "how would you like to have a plot here?"

Before I could answer, he stopped the car, got out and began walking toward the top of the hill.

"Look!" he said. "Wouldn't this be a nice place?"

"Yes," I said, "but must we pick out a lot today? It's Easter."

He walked back to the car and got in. He sat for a minute without switching on the engine.

"I wonder how expensive these lots are?" he said.

I knew from the size of the lot he had indicated that he wanted one big enough for three, for himself and me and Dan.

"Please, Woody," I said, "Can we go?"

My eyes blurred, and I thought I was going to cry. Hurriedly I looked away and wiped my eyes, hoping he didn't see the tears. If he did, he didn't mention them, but slowly drove back to the highway and turned toward the church.

We wound our way through some of the most beautiful apple-growing country in the world. The trees, blanketing the gently rolling hills, were almost bursting with blossoms. They filled the air with a fresh fragrance of goodness. We slowly drove the narrow road leading past the Bennetts, the Hootses, the Anderses, the Cases, the Hendersons, the Bakers, the Lappins, and finally the church parsonage where the Reverend Stanley and his family lived. Good, wholesome folks, these apple growers—salt of the earth, a special breed of people.

"How blessed we are," said Woody, "to live in such a beautiful part of the country."

Woody turned into the churchyard and drove slowly to the rear. He parked and got out with some effort, and walked slowly into the cemetery, reading the names on the grave markers. He didn't say a word, but I'm sure he was thinking that this was the place he would like to be buried. He wouldn't say it to me, however, because he thought I didn't want to place him in a country graveyard. Our membership was at the First Baptist Church in Hendersonville, but Tracy Grove is where we attended church through Dan's formative years. Because of Woody's great love for the outdoors, I had already decided that this is where he would be buried when he died. While he walked in the cemetery, the Smyths' rainbow-colored peacocks screamed in the distance, and an airplane droned far away. There were no other sounds, only the peace and quiet that the country produces.

We entered the chapel. It was small, filled with simplicity and heartfelt emotion. The congregation, dressed in Easter outfits, began to enter, slowly filling the chapel, and many came our way to say hello and wish us well.

Reverend Stanley and a deacon sat in the big chairs behind the pulpit, and Dale, the choir director, stepped forward with an open hymnal in his hand.

"Would you please turn your hymnals to page four-fifty-seven?" he said. His wife, Julia, was at the piano, and a girl from the community played the organ.

"Let's stand and sing," Dale said.

"Low in the grave He lay—Jesus, my Savior!" we sang. "Waiting the coming day—Jesus, my Lord! Up from the grave he arose...." I looked at Woody, and he was breaking up, tears streaming down his face. I took a tissue from my handbag and wiped his tears away, but he continued to cry through the entire service.

Although Woody wanted to be in church whenever he was able, he cried through all the services. This made it difficult for those sitting near him, but they were unsurpassingly patient, and their bodies throbbed with tenderness and compassion for Woody.

15

The middle of June was our family's time for vacations. My three brothers had made reservations for their families and us on a small island off the coast of South Carolina. Maurice lived in Maryville, Tennessee, and Leon and Jimmy lived in Woodruff, South Carolina. We had always gone vacationing together, making a big family gathering of it.

Because of Woody's condition, we felt we couldn't go, but my brothers knew how much we enjoyed the vacations, and they insisted that we come. I told them it would be impossible for us to work with Woody there, but my brothers adored him and refused to take no for an answer. They wanted Woody to enjoy everything as much as possible, and when they said they would not go without us, we agreed to go.

There would be four rented houses filled with relatives. Dan would take his girlfriend, Ann, along. She was a beautiful girl whom we liked a great deal.

On Thursday night and all day Friday, Dan and I packed everything we thought we would need. We had to take many additional things because of Woody.

It is hard to comprehend how much a man does around the house until he is incapacitated or no longer there. I did all the chores that were normally his responsibility, checking gas and oil for the car, and this and that. Woody reminded me of things to do, but could not lift a finger to help.

I worked late into the night, and was so exhausted I couldn't sleep, so I lay awake thinking. I should have had my tongue removed for ever having complained about anything in my life. I promised myself that as long as I lived, I would never grumble or express dissatisfaction about anything else. I had so much to be thankful for.

We planned an early start Saturday morning, and when the alarm rang, I jumped from bed. Dan left quickly to drive to Buies Creek in downstate North Carolina to pick up Ann, who was studying in summer school at Campbell College. We looked forward to having her with us on this vacation.

It was a beautiful day to travel. Woody felt good, and if we took our time, everything would be all right. His youthful face belied his forty-eight years, and the gray in his hair made him more handsome than ever. I was happy, yet sad, too, at the thought of such a beautiful man being so ill.

We brought a lunch so we could picnic on the way. That would be much easier than trying to get Woody in and out of a restaurant.

The day grew prettier as we drove down the mountains into South Carolina. Around noon, Woody spotted a roadside park and asked me to stop. We parked, took out the picnic basket, and chose a table at the back of the park, far away from the traffic. Huge pines towered around the table, and warm, brown pine needles crunched under our feet. The sun was warm, and its rays slanted through the trees. Dust particles floated in the shafts of sunlight and gleamed like gold.

Squirrels played around the tables, birds sang from almost every tree, a rabbit bounded across the highway toward us, and chipmunks talked with their friends. Above us, a red-headed woodpecker worked on a pine tree to get the insects inside the bark.

We had stopped in a lovely, cageless menagerie, and we had it all to ourselves—Woody and me and the animals.

During lunch, I began to worry. What if something happened to Woody here in the middle of nowhere? I didn't even know where the nearest hospital was. How foolish to travel alone with him! I urged him to hurry, but he wanted to stay longer, the place was so cheerful. Finally we finished and drove back onto the busy interstate. What a relief! We were back on the highway where I could get help if I needed it. "If we ever get safely to the beach," I told myself, "I'll never travel alone again."

In a few hours we were at the beach. Gorgeous clouds hovered over the ocean like huge white bags of cotton candy animals. We noted an elephant and a horse's head. Clouds at the beach always seem to be larger, brighter, and whiter than at home in the mountains. Today they were breathtaking.

We arrived at our cottage rather exhausted. Everything had been made ready for us; all we needed to do was relax and enjoy it. Woody was tired. "Let me help you out of the car," Jimmy said. I was surprised that Woody could even stand after so long a trip. He took short steps, methodically placing his walker, then one foot and the other, and so on.

We stopped at the porch to view the ocean. Waves splashed onto the beach, rolling in, flowing out, saying "Wel—come ... Wel—come!" Woody took a deep breath. "Boy," he said, "does that ever feel good." Then he began to cry. My brothers and their wives and children, waiting for Woody on the porch, began to cry, too.

This was just a sample, I knew, of what was in store for us this week. I was used to his crying, but the others were not, and I didn't know how it would affect them.

Woody said the first thing he wanted to do was buy about fifteen pounds of shrimp, cook them in a huge pot, and let everyone eat shrimp cocktail until they couldn't eat any more. And that's exactly what we did.

After dinner we all went down the walkway and sat watching the children play on the beach. Music blared and young people laughed in a small amusement park a block away, but we were too tired to go. The ocean was black as pitch, the sky, dark blue. Strange-looking crabs crawled everywhere. The tide was out, but still the waters rushed onto the sand with magnificent force.

Looking upon the waters and thinking of our home in the mountains, the words of Psalm 46: 1–3 came to me: "God is our refuge and strength, a very present help in trouble. Therefore will not we fear, though the earth be removed, and though the mountains be carried into the midst of the sea; though the waters thereof roar and be troubled, though the mountains shake. . . ."

Yes, I knew where my strength lay. And Woody's, too.

Before seven the next morning, Susie, Debbie, and Cheri knocked at our door, anxious to start the day. "Where do they get all that energy?" Woody asked, laughing.

That week was heavenly. Someone in the family was always with us, and we had little time to think about ourselves. The family had something planned every minute that Woody was able to be up. At times, even he forgot his illness.

Those were great days, Woody's last vacation. At night we played miniature golf. Woody could only hold the club in his left hand, but even handicapped he managed to beat us. Leslie, Mike, and Missie thought it was great that they could hold the club and place it in Uncle Woody's hand. The children had a deep, genuine compassion for Woody, surpassing that of most adults.

The nieces and nephews ranged in age from seven to eighteen, and they were like a three-ring circus that week, constantly laughing and joking and playing tricks on each other. Woody loved every minute of it.

Almost before we knew it, the week passed. With all the others on hand to watch Woody, I managed to rest well and relax that week.

We packed and left the beach. Jimmy and his wife Brenda drove behind us. Missie rode in the car to help with Uncle Woody.

The trip was trying, taking almost five hours to Woodruff where my parents lived. We stopped to rest and spend the night.

I helped Woody from the car. Thinking he was all right, I turned away for a moment, and he fell. The trip had drained him of his energy. But he didn't mind; he had had a wonderful week, and he knew this would be his last trip to the coast.

16

The week at the beach gave us a feeling of change, which we desperately needed, but now it was time to settle back into our routines.

The severity of Woody's affliction was oppressive. He was much harder to work with than even a month before. He felt the slightest wrinkle under his body. Anything out of place drove him up the wall. When I turned him in bed, I had to smooth out all the covers and check his pajamas for wrinkles. Regardless of how many pieces of lamb's wool we placed under him, he could still feel anything out of place. If anything, his sensitivity increased. He could not sleep until all the sheets and covers were smooth, then he sank into a state of complacency.

"The sheets feel like they weigh fifty pounds," he said.

I thought of using a bed cradle similar to those used in hospitals to keep the covers from being so heavy on his body. But a cradle would have to be moved each time I worked with Woody. I talked to my brother Leon, who owned a machine company in Woodruff, explaining an idea I had for a type of cover cradle that might work and would be less trouble.

Using conduit pipe, Leon and Jimmy made the cradle for me. They inserted the pipe between the mattress and the box springs at the foot of the bed, bent it upward to a point about a foot above the mattress, then ran it all the way to Woody's shoulders and across his chest, and back to the foot of the bed. I fastened the bed linen to the apparatus, and when I worked with Woody, all I had to do was push one pipe over, never disturbing the covers. The thing worked, and it made working with Woody a lot easier for me.

When the weather turned cold, we bought an electric queen-sized blanket, which completely covered the bed riser. I made sure that cold air couldn't seep in, and he slept comfortably, even on the coldest nights.

Woody could stand no weight on any part of his body. If I touched him, even holding his hand, I had to place his hand in mine, always with my hand on the bottom. Even putting my hand on his body drained him of the little strength he had left.

He could not stand to be closed up in a room. His bedroom was so far from the living part of the house that I moved him into a small room with windows on three sides that opened onto the patio. I painted the room a light green and placed his bed so he could see through all the windows. Through one, he could see the street, and see the neighbors go in and out, giving him something to think about other than himself.

One afternoon as I prepared dinner, Woody called me to turn him. As I worked with him he became extremely upset. I thought I had hurt him in some way. The more I worked, the more upset he became. He was looking beyond me toward the kitchen, his eyes bulging, but he was so upset he couldn't say a word. Suddenly, I smelled something burning. I wheeled and looked into the kitchen, and the stove was engulfed in flames. The pan on the stove had caught fire when I left.

I had too many irons in the fire!

I extinguished the flames quickly, but it took all after-noon to calm Woody. He was frightened of being trapped inside a burning house, but I assured him that if the house ever caught fire I would get him out if I had to drag him.

Late that night, after everything was quiet and settled, Woody called me to his bed.

"Barbara," he said, "will you hold me close and love me forever?"

I lay next to him, and I could feel the love being trans-mitted from his body to mine. He was unable to move, but his thoughts were powerful, so much so that he gained satisfaction just by my holding his body next to mine. The only way I could tell that he was making love to me was to look into his eyes. For a short time, his shackles were released, and he was temporarily freed from his prison.

He could drift off for a few minutes with me and for-get his problems. Then, almost as quickly as he drifted away, he would sink back into that horrible, invisible depth that so forcefully encased him. Once again, he had to fight to survive.

Months later, I learned that the muscles controlling our intimate life were the last to be destroyed. It breaks my heart to know there are thousands of paraplegics who are placed in hospitals to deteriorate gradually. Be-cause their bodies are degenerating doesn't mean they don't have the same feelings and needs they always had.

I determined that night that I would keep Woody at home until the last possible moment. I wanted him to spend as little time in the hospital as possible.

Releasing his emotional being was a way to relieve many of his frustrations, but it left me dangling in the air. I could take his arm and place it around my body, but it would only lie there like a piece of dead flesh. He could respond to me in thought, but couldn't as much as hold me close. I was an attractive woman in my late thirties who desperately needed to give love and to be loved. I could show him love, and I knew that he loved me. For me, there was a degree of satisfaction in that thought.

I remembered something I had written years ago: "Love is like beautiful green ivy that clings and holds with unbelievable strength. When old walls crumble under stress, beautiful green ivy quietly but surely creeps over the ruins and covers all the ugliness, and then there is beauty once more. . . ."

Would I ever have anyone to really love me again, and hold me close, the way I needed to be held? To think that only half of my life had been lived, and now Woody was going to die! I could feel the walls caving in. But I couldn't give up. I had to go on. He was such a great person. As long as he needed me, I would be there to do whatever I could.

17

One day Woody was walking about the living room with his cane, and he fell to the floor. I wrestled with him for fifteen minutes, trying to help him up.

When I got him back on his feet, I went to the kitchen for a glass of water—and heard another crash in the living room. Woody lay in the same spot as before.

"Woody," I said, "why didn't you stay in your chair?"

"Don't touch me," he said. "I can get up on my own. I don't need help."

For fifteen minutes, he worked around the coffee table and his chair, struggling to get up. His face became pale. Beads of perspiration rolled off his forehead, and I almost stepped in to help once or twice; but he was determined, and he managed to pull himself back into the chair.

He looked at me with a smile of triumph. His breathing was labored and his voice unsteady. "You see," he said, "I told you I could make it on my own. This illness is not going to lick me. I'll show you."

I only wished he could have been right. He knew as well as I that he was wrong, but for the moment it gave him encouragement.

It was impossible for me to maintain my composure that afternoon. To see him crawling on the floor like an animal almost killed me. By outward appearance, he was still a healthy-looking, handsome man, but a man with absolutely no strength. Tears welled into my eyes again.

I cried as hard as I had ever cried, and as I wept, Woody began apologizing for causing me all that trouble.

Imagine a man in his condition consoling me! That made me cry even harder. I could not control it.

It was one of the very few times through his illness that I fell apart, but I needed the cry in order to go on.

We had no way of knowing that that was to be the last time Woody would ever be able to get up off the floor without help.

18

With July came the hot, humid summer weather, and Woody's illness progressed. He had lost the use of both hands. I had to feed him all his meals. He still wanted to feed himself, but when he tried to move the spoon to his mouth, he spilled food into his lap. Getting through each meal was a painfully slow process.

He still attempted to use his walker, but with very little success. His legs were affected, and he fell more and more. Dan or I had to remain close by all the time. He resisted giving in to a wheelchair—he had unlimited determination, but, unfortunately, not enough muscular control to match. Using a wheelchair, he thought, would be an admission of defeat.

On a warm afternoon in mid-July, I placed Woody in the sunroom near the sliding glass door and went outside to work in my flowers. I cautioned him against trying to get up without calling me, because he was still in the stage when his mind would tell him he could do something, but his body would not respond. He would continually slip and try to do things behind my back, like a child.

I heard a loud crash behind me, and when I turned, I saw Woody lying with small shards of broken glass all over and around him. He had fallen into the glass door, and the entire pane had shattered into shrapnel-sized fragments.

Dan heard the crash, too, and came running. Woody lay in so much glass we were afraid to move him. I told Dan to get the vacuum cleaner and remove the fragments, and when we finally got him inside, I examined him carefully for cuts and abrasions. He had no swelling or pain, and I knew nothing was broken. His only injury was a half-inch cut on the back of his head.

Woody's brother Raymond, a minister who then served a church in Kernersville, North Carolina, near Winston-Salem, was visiting another brother, Andy, who lived in Hendersonville. Dan telephoned Raymond and told him of Woody's accident, and Raymond and Andy came over and replaced the pane.

From this time, I stayed with Woody constantly. I tried to convince him that he could no longer walk, that it was dangerous for him to try. Before this, we had talked mostly of things he could do; now I had to convince him there were things he could not do, without discouraging him to the point of giving up completely.

This was extremely hard for him to accept, but he finally gave in and let me do everything for him. He was experienceing progressive muscular atrophy. The illness had cut off all nourishment to the muscles and they were shrinking in size, gradually dying. He also agreed to use a wheelchair.

I found myself completely wrapped around Woody, never leaving him for more than a few minutes at a time. I became a prisoner, too, because the more I stayed with him, the more he came to depend on me. I became his only link to the world, watching every move he made, responding to all his requests.

I improvised things that would be useful to him. We had little money, so improvising became our way of life.

I propped an old television tray on one side of the kitchen table, and with two clothespins fastened the daily newspaper to the top of the tray. When I pushed Woody up to the table, he could read the paper by only asking me to turn the pages. He drank coffee or juice through a straw from a heavy-bottomed baby cup with a hole in the lid just large enough for a straw. I could prepare breakfast while Woody had juice and coffee and read the morning paper.

I could also fasten magazines and literature to the tray. It saved me quite a few minutes every day, and gave Woody many hours of pleasure.

I still had to keep an eye on him. Though he was unable to move his arms, he had a little strength left in his legs, and could move his body forward while sitting in his wheelchair. If he leaned too far forward, he fell out of the chair. To keep him from falling, I would lock his chair against the table while he had his meals.

As July wore into August, and August into September, Woody's deterioration became more noticeable day by day. Dan went back to school in September, and I wondered how much longer I could handle Woody alone.

Hospitalization, I knew, loomed nearer.

19

My brother Jimmy, and Brenda and their children, Mike and Melissa, visited us on a Sunday before Thanksgiving. All morning Woody talked about getting out for a short trip. He had been confined to the house for months, and the farthest he had gone was as far as I could push his wheelchair. My family knew this, and Jimmy and Brenda talked us into going home with them for a couple of days.

Getting ready for the trip was a painstaking and quite spectacular performance. The paraphernalia needed for Woody was unbelievable. I bathed Woody and dressed him, then we placed his wheelchair, bed cradle, bath riser, and other items in the car.

Jimmy and Mike packed the car, Brenda and Melissa talked with Woody, and I busied myself getting together the things we would need.

The phone rang. It was Dr. Lampley.

"What are you folks doing?" he asked.

I told him we were going out of town with Jimmy and Brenda.

"You can't do that," he said. "At least not for a couple of hours."

"Why not?"

"Because I have a surprise for you," he laughed. "I want to take you and Woody flying this afternoon."

It was a beautiful afternoon, brisk but not cold, and the sun moved across a cloudless sky.

I had no idea that Woody would go. Friends had invited us to go boating that summer, and he had refused. He had a fear of water and places that made him feel trapped. He couldn't even stand for me to buckle his seat belt in the car.

But when I told Woody of Dr. Lampley's request, he was thrilled, almost overwhelmed. He surprised me.

His adrenalin began pumping, and then a look of disappointment clouded his face.

"What's wrong?" I asked.

"How will I ever get in the plane?" he wondered.

Dr. Lampley was still on the line. I told him what Woody had asked, and he said, "Don't worry. I have four men standing by to lift him in."

"Then what are we waiting for?" Woody wanted to know.

We all drove to Winkler Aviation across town. Four men stood ready to lift Woody into the plane. He shivered as they put him inside. "Are you cold?" I asked.

"No," Woody said, "just a little nervous."

Dr. Lampley was a good pilot, but I was apprehensive—not for Woody, for once, but for myself. I could become queasy from turning my head the wrong way in a car, or by reading roadside signs. My stomach did flip-flops as we taxied down the runway and turned around.

Dr. Lampley revved up the engine, then released the brakes and gave the plane full throttle. We rolled down the runway, gathering speed, and then, with just the slightest quiver, rose into the air. He climbed gradually, and I watched the hangar slide away beneath us.

I turned to Woody, and he was smiling so broadly

there were tears in his eyes. He loved it! He laughed, but was so thrilled, he couldn't speak.

The flight was fantastic. We felt like kings of the world. Dr. Lampley pointed out places he knew that we would know—Jumpoff Mountain, Cold Mountain, the French Broad River, Pisgah and the Rat. The land rolled on and on beneath us, and we flew so high the farmlands appeared to be an old-fashioned fancy quilt that had been pieced together with hands of love and devotion. We flew over farms that had been handed down from generation to generation, groomed and worked and cared for as if they were priceless heirlooms. Suddenly I knew why this land was called "God's Country." God had fashioned it himself and lent pieces of it to us for a while.

Dr. Lampley pointed out a mountain cabin in which he and Woody and others had spent many nights while deer hunting. We saw deer grazing in broad fields that ran from one mountain to another.

Woody was so excited that I asked him repeatedly if he were all right. He shook his head yes; he still couldn't speak. We flew until dusk settled over the land. I felt a tranquility gently creep over me, and I thought of the thousands of families down below. Were they happy tonight? Would they go to bed tonight not realizing how fortunate they were to be able to walk and talk, even to move? I wanted to stand out on the wing and shout to them to be grateful. I wanted them to love each other, not to abuse friendships. Was this how God felt, looking down from above, seeing us going in all directions, knowing things could be different if we would only take the time to care? . . .

I was almost bursting with joy and love, and I wanted everyone to know God as I had come to know him, not as an ethereal being to whom we pay homage on Sunday morning, but as a living God who stands with us each day, in times of joy and sorrow, ready to help and advise, and always to give strength.

The sun slipped slowly behind the Great Smoky Mountains far ahead. They looked like a great herd of humpbacked buffalo grazing in the twilight. Mount Pisgah was a silhouette against a flaming sky to our left, and to the right, far away, the sun still glistened off Mount Mitchell, the highest peak east of the Rockies. What a lovely picture!

As we approached the airport, the runway lights were on, guiding us in. When the wheels lowered with a bump, I looked at Woody. His eyes were wide as silver dollars, and his voice began to return. I felt a wee bit nauseous, but it had been an incredible afternoon. When I stepped from the plane my feet were rubbery, but the flight had been one of the highlights of our winter.

The same four men were waiting to lift Woody from the plane. Mike and Melissa and Jimmy and Brenda stood at the gate, waving as if we had just returned from a long journey.

Jimmy helped put Woody in the car, and I drove our car behind Jimmy's down the mountains, around the curves, with the nausea still in me.

We fell into bed, exhausted. Woody slept for an hour, then awakened and called to me to turn him. He had to be turned thirty-five or forty times each night. In his sleep, Woody's mind would tell him he needed to be turned, but his body would not respond, and he would wake up and call to me. I slept very little those nights, four or five hours at the most. Before Woody's illness, my body had required eight to ten hours of sleep each night. I wondered how it was possible for me to work all day with him and stay up half the night, turning him.

We enjoyed our stay with the family in South Carolina, and after two days we returned home. I placed a small cot beside Woody's bed so I could sleep near him. I lost so much sleep I began to fear that I would sleep through his calls. A few times I did, and he became so frustrated that he stayed awake the rest of the night. How well we were able to rest depended on my turning him. During many nights, exhaustion overcame me to the extent that I had to crawl to his bed. Sometimes he needed only a finger or a leg moved, but he still had to wake me to do that.

He tried very hard not to disturb me, but it was more than he could handle. He differed from a paralyzed person in that he could feel everything.

He was compassionate, though. Each night before bed, he would say, "Barbara, I'll try not to disturb you tonight." And he did try, very hard, but the creature inside him was larger than the two of us. No matter how hard Woody fought, the creature always won.

I became even more determined. Regardless of how ill Woody became, he was going to live until the end. As long as I could drag myself, I was determined to care for him. Friends, and even relatives, cautioned me that I would destroy myself. Inside me, however, something said, "Keep going. You'll be all right."

Dan called several times each week to see how things were. I told him we were all right. I didn't want him to worry. I wanted him to stay in school. He always rang off by saying, "Mom, call me as soon as you need me."

At Christmastime, Dan came home for the holidays. When he walked into the house and saw how far his father had declined, he was shocked. He immediately telephoned his school and withdrew for the remainder of the semester. He drove back to school, gave up his apartment, and moved his things home. In six months he would have graduated, but he didn't hesitate.

"Nothing," he told me, "is as important as taking care of you and Dad."

Dan immediately started learning all the techniques of caring for his father. He observed Woody in the same fashion that I had done, learning everything he could. If I die, I thought, Dan will be able to care for Woody.

We tried every day to do all we could to make Woody's life easier. We gave him exercise three times a day, holding him in a standing position against the wall and moving his limbs for twenty minutes. This kept his blood circulating, and helped prevent bedsores.

By coming home, Dan prolonged his father's life—and possibly saved mine.

We didn't have time to do our Christmas shopping until 4 o'clock Christmas Eve. Soon after we returned, Dr. Lampley and his parents came by with Christmas presents. Later, Coy Robertson dropped in with his daughter April and son Steve, the Holden girls, and little Danny, with whom Woody played when he shut Dan and me out of his life. The children had made fruit baskets for Woody, and they sang carols.

Considering the circumstances, it was a nice Christmas.

20

Sunday morning, January 15, 1975, dawned cold and rainy. It would be the longest morning of Woody's illness, at least for me. It was the day we would take him to the hospital, never to return home. We didn't know that at the time, but we suspected it.

Woody had been ill for almost two years, and his nerves had been shot for longer than that. Though we had talked many times about hospitalization, it didn't make it easier for Woody. He was extremely nervous. He felt as if he were facing a whole new life in his thoroughly weakened condition.

Dan and I gave him a shower that morning, and he began to cry.

"Don't cry, Woody," I said, "We'll take care of you. We'll never leave you."

He had almost lost the power of speech, but he cut his eyes toward me and said, "I'm okay. Don't worry." He continued to cry. He couldn't help it. We were as accustomed to his crying as anyone can get; he cried several times each day—but today it was hard for Dan and me to hold back our own tears.

The doctors had told us that he would have involuntary outbursts of laughing and crying, that it was caused by damage to higher nuclear centers above the brain stem. When I asked Woody why he was crying, he would say, "Don't worry about me. I can't help crying."

Dan and I learned to know when he was happy and when he was sad, and we could tell when his crying was involuntary and when it wasn't. That helped us tremendously.

Margaret R. Pardee Hospital was only four blocks from our home. Dr. Lampley had made all the arrangements; all we had to do was get ready to go. Dr. Lampley knew it would be a hard day for us. He was always there, helping every way he could to make our lives easier.

Once, three months before, I had sought an electric bed for Woody, but couldn't find one. Dr. Lampley called.

"Barbara," he said, "I told you if you needed anything to call me. Now what kind of bed do you want?"

I told him the type bed we wanted, and early the next morning he knocked on our door and had the bed with him. I learned later that he had been up all night with a young man who had lost his arm in a plant accident. But he cared enough to help us, even under those extreme circumstances.

When we were ready to leave for the hospital, my father warmed up the car. He and Mother had come over early that morning to help us.

"It's cold outside," Woody said. Dan wrapped a wool blanket around the wheelchair. I said, "Don't worry. Don't worry." I could find no other words.

We put Woody in the car, and he slowly looked at the house and lawn as if making a mental photograph. I almost knew that he felt he would never see the house again.

Rain pelted harder against the windshield as we drove to the hospital. The cold was penetrating.

"Looks like snow," my father said.

Woody began to cry. "I'd like to see it snow one more time," he said. That's the closest he ever came to mentioning his impending death.

I tried to console him about entering the hospital, for I knew he was afraid.

"Maybe we'll be able," I said, "to take leaves of absence and come home for weekends."

He did not respond.

We arrived at the hospital, one bag, one wheelchair, and Woody. Dan pushed him up the ramp to the emergency entrance. I held his hand. My mother and father were close behind.

The place, like most hospitals, looked cold. Bells rang, the intercom blared for doctors, people hurried in all directions. We came to the admitting office. Eliner King, whom we have known for years, was at the desk. She is a lovely lady who always makes you feel better.

"Hi, Woody," she said. "So good to see you. I've made all the arrangements for you and Barbara." What a fantastic service she did for Woody that day! Her kindness meant so much to him.

He looked at her and smiled. "Thank you," he said.

She snapped a bracelet on his wrist, patted his hand, and said, "Okay, we're ready to go upstairs. Wait just a minute, and I'll take you."

Woody's tears began to flow. I wiped them away. We didn't dare say much—actually, we couldn't, not without breaking down ourselves. People in the hall stared at us. They didn't understand that Woody could not control his emotions, but I could feel the palpitation of the heartaches in their bodies.

After several minutes, Mrs. King returned. She patted Woody on the shoulder. "Okay, Woody," she said, "we're ready to go."

I stepped to one side, and Dan turned the wheelchair

around. My father picked up the little black valise and carried it in his right hand. I caught my mother's arm. She glanced at me with a gentle smile of genuine love and took my hand and held it close. I was forty, but still her little girl.

We walked down the hall, following the wheelchair, and came to the door of the tiny chapel. I looked at the stained glass at the back, and we paused for a moment to give thanks to God for his continued strength in our struggle.

I have open communication with God. I don't ask for specific things. I feel that if God knows every hair on our heads, he knows our needs. In all of Woody's illness, we had never asked God to heal him, nor had we asked for anything for ourselves except the strength to continue. We had asked that God's will be done in our lives.

Woody prayed within himself. Many times I had seen him sitting on the patio or the wall beside the garden with his eyes closed, and I knew he was communicating with God.

It's so simple to communicate with God; *we* make it hard.

The chapel was undersized, giving it an appearance of unimportance, yet at the same time it exuded a feeling of assuagement. A dozen chairs were lined up undisturbed along two walls. The room appeared to have never been occupied, and, indeed, as many times as I had been there, I had never seen anyone in that room. The stained glass pane in the rear of the room gave an illusion of candle-light, and the feeling came over me that this was a unique and very special place. For the next ten months, I would sit quietly in this room many times.

Mrs. King halted Woody at the elevator door and waited for us. My father stepped into the elevator first and held the door for Dan to roll Woody in. A sign in the elevator announced a bloodmobile location, and that turned my thoughts back to Woody. He was a gallon donor. He had given blood six months before his illness was diagnosed. I wondered who had received his blood and whether his illness could be transmitted that way.

My father appeared to be calm, but he had a nervous cough that always told on him. Hack, hack, hack! He had coughed all morning.

Woody looked up at me. "I'm okay," he said.

"I know, Woody," I said. "God is taking care of us."

Mrs. King walked to the nurses' station. "We are supposed to go to Two-B," she said to a nurse with dark, curly hair. The nurse rose to lead us down the hall.

We passed a room with a sign on the door that read, "Caution! No Smoking! Oxygen!" I looked in and could see a small, mummylike figure under the taut white sheet. She lay very still. Her face was that of an old woman. Someone's grandmother was dying, I thought.

The dark-haired nurse turned her eyes toward me as if to say, "Keep going!"

My mind began to wander. The nurse was a warden, Woody a prisoner being punished for a crime he didn't commit! He was strapped in his wheelchair, unable to move. There were no doors, no way out, the windows barred. Each door was closed and locked behind us. There was no escape, no hope!

We screamed to the nurses for help. "Don't you understand? We need help. He is being punished for a crime he didn't commit!"

I heard only the echo of my own voice. Woody was doomed! And no one cared!

"Barbara." I heard the voice as if it were coming from deep in a well. "Barbara!"

It was Mrs. King. She looked at me strangely. I snapped back. "I'm sorry," I said. "I think I was dreaming."

We were in Woody's room across the hall from the

nurses' station. His good friend, Marian Hines, was in charge that day, and she had everything ready.

"I want you near the station, Woody," Mrs. Hines said, "so we can keep an eye on you."

He smiled.

"We'll give you the best of care."

He began to cry.

"Thank you," he said through the tears, and then he really choked up.

Mrs. Hines walked out of the room. She knew we could calm Woody.

The spotless bed with sheets tightly stretched had been freshly made for Woody. I wondered who had slept there before. Had the patient died? Would Woody die in that bed? When? These questions crept through my mind.

Was Woody thinking the same thing?

We were so tuned in to each other. I turned away to keep him from reading my thoughts.

We had requested a private room, but there were none available. A man who had had surgery lay in the bed by the window, his wife at his bedside. I introduced myself to them, then introduced Dan and Woody. They were nice people.

We didn't object to a double room, but the presence of another patient in the room, I thought, might jeopardize what we had toiled so long to attain. Woody had been promised the first available private room, but after two days the other patient was discharged, and no one else was moved in.

As I put Woody's things in the bedside table, I thought, "You come into this world with nothing, and you surely go out of it with nothing."

All he had were two pairs of pajamas, a small shaving kit, a tooth brush, a pair of slippers, a beautiful red robe, and forty-eight years of memories.

Dan worked with Woody, who always needed something scratched or rubbed. Today his nose was itching and Dan rubbed it.

Woody became tickled, and couldn't stop laughing. The man in the other bed began to chuckle, and his wife smiled.

Woody's laughter suddenly turned to tears. He gasped with uncontrolable weeping. Dan and I petted him, trying to calm him. The other man and his wife must have thought we'd all flipped our lids. I must have looked like a possessive mother caring for a child, but looks didn't matter.

No one on the floor had seen an ALS patient. This would be a new experience for them. If they could spend time with Woody and observe the illness, and observe the tremendous growth mentally and spiritually, it would be rewarding; but, of course, they had many patients, and their time was limited.

I wouldn't give the time I had spent caring for Woody for all the riches of the world. It brought to my life many hours of satisfaction and gratification.

We put Woody's bright red robe on him to avoid the chill that this new experience gave him. I had made the robe for him. He looked great in red; it added color to his cheeks. Since his illness began, I had dressed him in bright colors—red, yellow, blue—and they helped keep up his spirit. He loved to look good, though he usually felt bad.

The afternoon passed, and night came on. My parents had left in midafternoon. Dan and I stayed.

I had had little rest for months, and a severe case of nerves infested my body. Woody and I had talked about this before he entered the hospital, and he had hoped that his being hospitalized would permit me to be away for a few hours each day. I had hired a licensed practical nurse to be with him that first night to see how things went. Before hiring her, I talked with her on the phone, explaining how difficult it was to work with an ALS patient. Her name was Mrs. Freeman, and she seemed more than willing to work with us.

I waited for her at the door with anticipation and devout feelings of emotional surrender. I had not been away from Woody, and I had mixed emotions about leaving. I felt I was abandoning him when he still needed me. But I also knew his illness was going to destroy, and I wasn't sure at this point whether it would destroy Woody or me first.

Whatever, I had no choice. I needed rest.

As I waited at the door, I saw a fairly large woman appear around the corner, carrying a large tote bag and some books. She had a brace on her leg and walked with a slight limp. She came straight to Woody's room.

"Hello," she said. "I'm Ella Freeman."

"I know," I said. "I felt it was you when you turned the corner."

I was so relieved that she was willing to work with us, and that she was a nice, pleasant woman, that I hugged her.

"Woody," I said, "this is Mrs. Freeman."

"Thanks for coming," he said. "I know your son and daughter-in-law."

He began to cry.

"Can you understand him?" I asked. He slurred his words now.

"Yes," Mrs. Freeman said. "I think so. Just give me a few nights. We'll be fine, won't we, Woody?"

She talked loudly, as though she thought he had a hearing problem. Most people talked to him that way. Because his body had deteriorated, they thought his hearing was impaired. Some even thought his mind was affected.

I explained to her that there was nothing wrong with his hearing, that he was a complete man, but without any strength.

Woody grinned. "That's right," he said.

I settled Woody down, and explained everything about him that I could think of to Mrs. Freeman. At midnight I left the hospital with a melancholy feeling in my heart.

When I reached home, I fell across the bed, feet dangling off one side, arms off the other, hoping to rest for a moment. I fell into a deep sleep, still dressed.

21

The ringing of the telephone woke me at 11 o'clock the next morning. I was still dressed; I had slept in my clothes.

"Mrs. Shelton?" the caller inquired. "This is Mrs. Clark at the hospital. Woody needs you at once!"

"What's wrong?"

"I don't know. We can't understand him."

I threw myself together and drove quickly to the hospital. He can't void, I thought. He had not been able to void in bed since his illness began. We always helped him to the bathroom and held him.

When I rushed into his room, he said, "I wanted you to get some rest, but I can't make it without you." He spoke haltingly, slurring his words. He was difficult to understand.

An orderly had sat him on the side of the bed and turned him loose, and it frightened him. Woody tried to tell the orderly that he could not sit alone, but the orderly could not understand. All Woody could make him understand was to call me. Everyone at the hospital was so kind and gentle to him, but ALS was so new to them that it would take time for them to learn to care for Woody. In the meantime, I would have to stay with him all day.

He kept repeating, "Tell them never to turn me loose."

I spent that day getting him adjusted to his new home. He felt safe in the hospital. He thought they might have some answers for him, but, of course, they didn't. No one did. It was still up to us.

He now had trouble swallowing. He choked a lot and was afraid he might choke to death. He felt safer with doctors and nurses around, but didn't want me to leave even then.

Dr. Lampley gave me permission to use the aspirator on Woody. My training as a dental assistant came in handy then. I knew the proper way to suction, and didn't come unglued when I had to do it.

That night we decided to have Mrs. Freeman again. She was a delightful lady in her sixties. At first I thought she might resent my telling her so much about the illness. After all, she was a nurse, and I wasn't. But she was quite anxious to learn all the techniques I could teach her.

Woody adored her from the minute she walked into the room. He felt at ease and comfortable with her. Each afternoon he gave me his requests, and when she came on duty I would go over them with her. I had worried about getting a nurse for him because of all the work involved and his strict requirements. He demanded that he never be left alone. That, in itself, was enough to scare some LPNs away, but not Mrs. Freeman. I told her that before she came, and she was still game.

Since she wore a leg brace for some kind of arthritis, I was apprehensive. I didn't know if she could stand up under all the strain, and I didn't wish the job to make her sick. But she felt good about working with Woody, and I knew God had sent her into our lives at a time when I didn't think I could hold up much longer.

Woody had to be turned six or eight times every half-hour. I had a way of turning him that differed from the way the nurses had been taught, and my way was more comfortable to him since he was used to it. Mrs. Freeman was more than willing to turn him my way. His body had become so fragile that I was afraid of fracturing his bones. He was no more than a bag of bones with a little flesh and skin stretched over them. The doctors had told us that the illness would destroy all of Woody's voluntary muscles, but it seemed to me that it eventually destroyed the involuntary ones, too.

Turning Woody, I would take a handful of pajama at the hip and a handful at the shoulder, and with a gentle pull toward me, roll him up and over on his side. Then I bent the bottom leg at the knee, and did the same with the top leg. I had made little foam pillows to stuff between his knees, and I put his top foot behind his bottom foot. He could not stand the weight of one foot on top of the other. Finally, I pulled his arm out from beneath his body, and put the top arm over the bottom arm, never letting them touch.

As I worked with each part of the body, I asked him if it was comfortable. When finished, I looked at his body and asked myself if I would be comfortable in that position. If he were comfortable, he would smile and go to sleep. If not, he would remain awake until I found the uncomfortable limb.

He worked with eye language. I would tell him, "Close your eyes if. . . ." If it was right, he would close his eyes; if not, he would keep them open. I started all questions to him with "Close your eyes if. . . ." For the present, this worked rather well, but I knew that I would need to work out a better method soon.

22

It was most important to find ways for Woody to speak as he progressed from one stage of illness to another. A sense of frustration and alienation resulting from a breakdown in communication can result in psychological damage, and we wanted to avoid that.

We rarely pause to appreciate our privilege of communication. So many people talk so much and say so little—they speak, but they don't communicate. Many couples communicate only briefly between mouthfuls of food, or during television commercials—and they miss so much.

One of the truly sad parts of Woody's illness was his loss of speech. As his body withered away, his mind remained clear. He could not move, and he could not talk, yet he was aware of everything that went on around him. That's why I had to come up with a device that would enable him to communicate.

I thought about communication for days and finally worked out an ABC board. I divided the alphabet into five lines on a large, white sheet of paper, and holding the paper at Woody's eye level and watching his eyes, I began.

"Start at the beginning of the first line," I told him. "If the letter you want is in that line, blink your eyes. If not, we'll move to the second line, and so on."

When he came to the right letter, he would close his eyes, and I would write the letter down. The method necessitated two blinks for each letter, one for the proper line, the other for the letter.

The method was slow, but it worked. Sometimes it would take fifteen or twenty minutes to find out what he wanted, but working the board not only enabled him to communicate, it also gave him something constructive to do with his time. Idle time was his enemy.

One reason he became so proficient in using the ABC board, I think, is because we devised it and practiced on it before he entirely lost his speech. He could say only a few words, and I could barely make them out. We worked with the board constantly, and the more we worked, the more comfortable he became. He seemed to know that I would find ways to help him. God gave me the answers to many of his needs. Also, working with him constantly helped keep his spirits up and reassured him that we would never leave.

One afternoon a nurse from physical therapy came in with Dr. Lampley.

"Woody," the doctor asked, "would you like a nice soak in the Hubbard tub?"

Woody's eyes got large as silver dollars. "I . . . don't . . . know," he said, looking at me for help. I knew he was thinking he might be left alone.

"I'll go with you," I said.

He agreed. Anne Stoneman was one of the therapists, Darrell Rhodes was the other. Woody and I had known Anne from years back. Her husband had died, leaving her with five small children. She did a wonderful job in rearing them.

Rhodes was a tall, quiet man who spoke with a gentle, warmhearted tone. Anne was also quiet, extremely kind, and very pretty.

"Is it all right if I stay?" I asked Anne.

"Of course it is," she said. She looked at Woody. "Are you ready to go swimming?" she asked, smiling.

"I . . . guess," Woody said.

He was apprehensive, but willing to try anything that might help him. Anne adjusted things around the tub, and Woody was placed on a stretcher. As they lowered him into the tub, he almost lost his breath. Anne was patient in adjusting him to the water gradually.

When he was immersed, Anne left the room to work with another patient. The stretcher was tilted feet down into the water, and Anne had placed a towel under his arms and neck to keep his head out of the water. Though he was strapped to the board, he kept sliding down because he had no muscles with which to hold himself back. I held him in place and got him to relax.

He enjoyed the bath. He laughed and cried. The water must have felt good to him, circulating with a bit of pressure.

After the bath, Anne took us back upstairs. She wanted to see if he could walk, thinking the exercise might be good for him. I thought he was trying to do too much in one afternoon, but he felt so good after the bath that he didn't want to stop. With two persons holding him up and helping him place one foot ahead of the other, he was able to walk a few steps.

Back in bed, Woody felt fine—for an hour. He was completely relaxed and a bit heady over his accomplishments. After an hour, however, his entire body began to ache, and for several days he was so fatigued that he could barely breathe.

When he began to recover, he asked for the ABC board, and spelled out: "Tell them I don't want any more baths." I went to the head nurse and cancelled all his bath appointments.

Mrs. Freeman worked out remarkably well. Each night at 11:30 I was at liberty to leave the hospital and tend to my own needs. Woody was comfortable with Mrs. Freeman, who took exceptional care of him. But I had to be back in the hospital early each morning to be with him when Mrs. Freeman went off duty.

One morning when I came into Woody's room, a young man whom I hadn't seen before was with him. His name was Gary Musselwhite. He was a student at a nearby Seventh-day Adventist nursing school which brought students to the hospital regularly to work with patients and get on-the-floor experience. Gary had been assigned to Woody for a week.

Haltingly, Woody said, "Barbara . . . this is . . . Gary. He's from . . . Mountain San." In a moment, he added, "Is . . . he . . . ever . . . great!"

I could see the moment I walked in that Gary was indeed great. He was twenty-one, more than six feet tall, had dark, curly hair and blue eyes. He wore white trousers and a blue jacket, and his voice was musical and soothing.

Gary was just what Woody needed, a male to work with him and talk with him, and before the end of the week, Woody and I knew that Gary had answered his calling. He was cut out to be a male nurse. He was so good with Woody that by the end of the week we were ready to adopt him as our second son. After that week, until Woody's death, Gary visited him every time he had an opportunity.

When the doctors saw that Woody's stay in the hospital might be lengthy and that he had adapted well to hospital life, they arranged for him to be moved into the Lane Wing, the hospital's extended care facility.

His new room was like one in the Holiday Inn. The extended care facility was about two years old, the room was rather large and clean and fresh, the way a hospital should be. The room had a walk-in shower, a television set, a large dresser with mirror, and a small window at one side. The mirror had a recessed light at the top, and I kept fresh flowers in front of it with the light shining on them. Outside the window was a small garden with loads of greenery. The room was a lovely place to care for a long-term patient.

By then, Woody could move nothing except his eyes and his right big toe. Since the nurses could no longer see from their station directly into his room, I tried to think of a way to rig a call button that Woody could use if he needed help at any time I was out of his room. I talked to the head nurse about it, and I asked if she could have a maintenance man visit us.

Late that afternoon, Vance Frady, a maintenance man, came in, and we talked about an improvised call button.

"Let's see if we can rig one he can press with his toe," Frady said.

With epoxy, he glued a piece of wood, like a bar, to a regular call button. This he mounted on a 15-by-25-inch board, and placed the board upright at the foot of Woody's bed in such position that Woody could touch the bar with his toe and ring for a nurse. The board could be removed from the bed and placed on the footboard of Woody's wheelchair.

Each time I left the room, I placed his toe on the call button. All he had to do was press it to call the nurse.

Frady also rigged a television control onto the board, and Woody could turn the TV on and off and change channels with a touch of his toe.

Woody and I played silly games. Outside our room we built an imaginary porch, and every day we imagined sitting on the porch for hours, talking to everyone who came by. Sometimes another patient would come to see

Woody and he, too, would sit on the porch and play the game with us.

Woody didn't have a lot of company because, in his condition, he cried every time someone came in, which not only upset Woody, but his visitors as well. Friends still maintained telephone contact with us and stood by ready to help in any way, but their visits were infrequent, and then they usually just popped in to say hello and went on their way.

A few continued to visit anyway, whether Woody cried or not—Dale and Julia Lappin, Coy Robertson, Ernie Dezzutto, Stella Langton, Aunt Ressie. Dr. Barber came each Wednesday afternoon. They brought flowers and gifts, and especially made Valentine's Day and the Fourth of July bearable by giving Woody parties in his room.

Occasionally a nurse would be a little gruff with Woody, and this cut him to the bone. But I knew that this was a way she coped with the dying. It is difficult to be around people who die a bit each day.

23

Lane Wing was a forty-bed unit, and many of the beds were filled with the dying or senile. Woody was about the youngest and, unquestionably, the most handsome. We made many friends. Patients in Lane Wing came to be members of one big family.

Late each afternoon, after dinner, I pushed Woody down the hall to a large lounge, and Blanche and Maudine were always there waiting for someone, usually another patient, to come for a visit.

Maudine was an attractive lady in her middle forties, afflicted with multiple sclerosis. She had warm, brown hair and bright eyes. She could not hold a pen to write and had no control over her bladder. She could only move her right arm as far as her mouth, and she was not able to perform the most minute tasks. She couldn't brush her teeth or comb her hair and apply makeup.

Blanche, in her sixties, was also a friendly woman who had a disease that rendered her body useless.

Each time I saw them, I thanked God for my own health and strength. As we talked and shared with Maudine and Blanche, my heart knew a gnawing ache of sympathy. I wanted so much to reach out and touch them and tell them they would be well.

My mind raced again with questions. What if I were in

Maudine's place? Or Woody's, or Blanche's? What if I could not move to comb my hair or fix my face? What if no one came to visit or help me? What if I had to stay in the hospital day after day, week after week, month after month? Could I stand it? There was such need for those healthy people around them to take time just to talk and share a few thoughts, but few noticed. They didn't realize, those healthy creatures didn't, that at any moment they could be stricken like Woody or Maudine or Blanche.

Those who are afflicted learn to love and give and share and hold onto every precious moment with every ounce of strength they have remaining. Woody's illness had certainly educated Dan and me. We learned that there are two worlds: One you can measure with line and rule, and another you can feel with your heart and imagination.

The hospital walls were thin, and day after day as Woody's body continued to deteriorate, his hearing improved. He could often hear the nurses at their station talking. Sometimes they discussed the condition of other patients, sometimes they discussed Woody. Often their words brought tears to his eyes. So his room became both a heaven and a hell.

Woody's main concern became his nerves, and he constantly wanted me to explain that to the nurses. "I hope they understand my nerves can't stand any problems," he spelled out on the ABC board one day. The nurses were our close friends, many of them we had known for years, and if one was too busy or too involved to stop and speak to Woody, he would look at me with desperation and grief in his eyes. He had the emotions of a child who had been punished in error.

By March of 1975, Woody had lost all interest in television, nor did he desire to be read to from newspapers and magazines. His nerves were at the breaking point. He was so edgy, he couldn't stand for me to read the newspaper to myself; the rustling of the pages bothered him. That 14-by-14 room grew smaller each day.

Dan came faithfully every afternoon to stay with his father, but even so, Woody didn't want me out of his sight. He thought that if I left him in the daytime, something would detain me, and he would be in trouble. Each time I had to leave, he would ask for the talk board and spell out, "Hurry back," or "Don't stay long."

By late spring, he could no longer hold up his head. When we put him in his wheelchair, his head dropped over on his shoulder, or his chin fell to his chest. We tried a neck collar without much success, and finally I drove to Asheville and rented a reclining wheelchair. By reclining him to a ninety-degree angle, he could sit comfortably without the neck collar. I made a small pillow to support his head, and placed a two-inch foam pad beneath his buttocks.

His hands, however, continually fell off the arm rests and dangled beside the chair. One morning, I let my own arms dangle off the sides of my chair, and after ten minutes pain stabbed through my arms to my elbows.

I got the ABC board and asked Woody if his hands and arms hurt when they dangled. "Yes," he spelled out, "almost all the time when they hang like this." Without the talk board, we never would have known.

Dan cut a seven-inch board the width of the wheelchair, and each morning I wrapped a hospital towel around the board and placed it on his chair before him. We positioned his hands on the board, giving him much relief.

After that, when I asked if his hands and arms hurt, he spelled "No."

That spring, Woody sat at his window every day and

watched a pair of robins build a nest in a tree. The male had a bright, orange-red breast. His neck was brownish gray, his head black. His outer tail feathers were tipped with white. What a beautiful bird! The female was smaller and duller in color.

The female built the nest with occasional help from the male. She formed a cup-shaped structure from bits of roots, string, paper, and twigs, cemented it together with mud, and lined it with dried grass. Soon after that, their young hatched, and then both of the parents busied themselves carrying food to their newborn.

We talked of the old English legend about the bird that mercifully picked a thorn from the crown of Christ as he carried the cross to Calvary, and as the bird carried the thorn in its beak, a drop of blood fell to its breast, dyeing it red. That was the robin.

For weeks after that, we could hear the robins singing, "Cheerily, cheerily." They didn't have a care in the world. They seemed to sense that we were just inside, but they were not afraid.

By May, Woody's nerves were so frayed he could no longer stand to see anyone, not even members of our families. Until then, his family and mine had visited him regularly, coming from all across the states. He asked Dan and me to explain that he loved them and would like to see them, but couldn't. Woody's family, especially, was scattered. Raymond lived in Kernersville, Chester in Columbus, Ohio, Roy in Cincinnati, Dorothy in Washington Courthouse, Ohio, Mabel in Santa Cruz, California, Ines in Barbersville, West Virginia. Andy was the only brother who lived in Hendersonville.

Anytime Woody saw anyone, he went into hysterics and choked and coughed until I thought he would die.

It took both Dan and me to turn him, one to do the turning, the other to hold his head. We felt that the slightest bobble could break his neck, and we reached the point where one of us stayed with him every minute of the day, and a nurse stayed at night. We didn't leave him for a minute.

Feeding him became more and more a problem. He could no longer handle a bite as large as a baby bite. When he drank from a straw, he could pull the fluid only halfway up. With scissors I cut his straws in half, and he managed. He drank food supplements through the straw. His intake of food fell to almost nothing, and his body became so thin and frail that you could see every bone.

He had to rely more and more upon valium and sleeping medication, and often he had trouble opening his eyes. It became difficult for him to use the talk board, and Mrs. Freeman had trouble communicating with him at night.

I made signs of his most needed requests—"hot," "cold," "water," "call Barbara"—and put them on the wall. When he was unable to get Mrs. Freeman to understand his needs, he would look toward the signs, and she would touch each in turn until she came to the right one, and he would weakly close his eyes.

Finally, Mrs. Freeman had to leave the job. She had performed wonderfully well and had become a friend. Audrey Moore, a lovely, gray-haired lady in her sixties, helped us for several weeks. She was kind and gentle with Woody. But she, too, had to leave.

Betty Stevenson, a capable young woman in her thirties, took the job, and immediately fell in love with Woody. Everyone who worked with him came to love him. Betty worked every night except Saturday. She needed Saturday night to be with her family for the weekend.

So Saturday became my night to stay, and I was able to alternate it with Gary Musselwhite. Ann Aiken, Dan's girl friend, spent that summer in Hendersonville, and she helped with Woody a couple of hours each day, so that I could get away.

We were fortunate to have such people who cared for Woody and who were willing to work with him. I think God sent them into our lives.

Through the summer, Woody experienced a lot of discomfort. His condition grew gradually worse. Dan and I reached the point where we could read Woody's thoughts. We knew without looking when he needed us. We felt his need for something before he asked.

In August, he lost control of his bowels, but his bladder still functioned. He received daily enemas. By September, he almost stopped eating. My mother cooked and pureed foods for him at home, but he had trouble ingesting.

We asked for him to be moved back to Two-B, where he would be watched closer, and he was moved into a double room from which one of the beds had been removed. Two large windows overlooked Jumpoff Mountain, and from his bed Woody could look at the mountain. He spent little time in his wheelchair, though we still tried to take him for a short ride each day. Before that, we had ridden him down the halls several times a day.

By September, he was experiencing a lot of pain. One day a tremendous pain entered his chest. He wanted to scream, but couldn't. He spelled out for me to call the doctor. An examination and X rays showed that he had developed a pulmonary embolism, and he was put on powerful antibiotics. For fourteen days he was fed intravenously.

We thought he would surely die, but he pulled through the crisis, and soon he wanted to get up and go for rides again. He laughed and talked on the board. His brother and sister-in-law came to see him, and he enjoyed them. He could see close friends again, but he still broke up at the sight of most members of the family.

Once, however, he asked to see Jimmy and Brenda and their children. I telephoned Jimmy, and he drove his family up immediately. The nurses arranged for the children to come up the back way because they were too young to be admitted as regular visitors, and Woody was delighted to see them. They stayed for an hour. Seeing Mike and Melissa gave him a lift.

Each morning when I went into Woody's room, Betty Stevenson would say how exhausted she was, and I kept saying, "Oh, if only you can hold on just a little longer." And she did. She was a Trojan. She was so good with Woody that if anything happened to her at this point, with the real communication problem we had with Woody, I didn't know what I would do.

Even she had trouble understanding everything he wanted during the night. His medication was stronger, and he was often so sedated that he couldn't lift his eyelids.

I walked into his room one morning, and he wanted his talk board immediately. He spelled out that when Betty had turned him last, his head was pushed a little far and he had difficulty breathing. He wanted me to tell her to always ask him if he needed his head pushed back. When she came to work that evening, I told her, and she said he seemed to be uncomfortable, but that she couldn't determine why.

24

On the fifteenth of November, Woody spelled out on the board that his jaws were locked and he could not swallow. From that time on, he never took any food through the mouth, not even a teaspoon of water. He told me on the board that the pain was excruciating. He began taking morphine and heavier injections of sleeping medication. He asked for it during the day.

One night, during the last week of Woody's life, he asked me to call his brother Raymond and tell him to come. I told Woody I would call Raymond in the morning. "No," he spelled out. "Call him now." I telephoned, and Raymond said he would come early the next morning. "Tell him," Woody spelled out, "to come now."

At midnight, Raymond arrived. He had driven almost two hundred miles. He prayed with Woody, and Woody roused up enough to talk with Raymond, using the talk board, of course. The visit meant much to Raymond, who had not been able to see Woody since spring. He loved Woody very much, as did the whole family.

Raymond stayed with Dan and me for a week.

On another evening that week, Dan and I found ourselves at home for a short while together. He sat in a chair, playing his guitar, and I lay on the floor, trying to relax. Suddenly Dan stopped playing, and said, "Mom, do you feel that feeling in the room?"

"What do you mean, Dan?"

"When I walk down the hall and come to Dad's room, I feel we're encased in a bubble, like there is a higher power in there, taking care of us."

"That's quite strange," I said. "I've felt that for some time, but didn't know anyone else did."

The next morning when I got to the hospital, I kissed Woody and sat on his bed and told him about what Dan and I had discussed. Woody wanted his talk board, and he spelled out, "I have felt that for many months."

We all had that special feeling that God was looking out for us, protecting us.

Woody was down to eighty pounds. He had not had a haircut for a long time, and I couldn't shave him frequently because it made him uncomfortable. Fortunately, he didn't have a heavy beard.

Dr. Lampley was out of town, but he telephoned every day to ask how Woody was.

Woody's pain grew worse, and that day it became so bad that I asked the head nurse to call Dr. Sellers. He came in five minutes, examined Woody, and worked with him.

I said to the doctor, "I don't understand why he is asking for so much pain medication now. He's been in pain for months, but he hasn't been asking for this much medicine before."

Dr. Sellers said, "This may be his way of wanting out of the whole thing. He's thinking that when he's asleep, he's all right."

Dr. Sellers came every day that week. He was there when we needed him. He talked with Woody, he examined him, and he gave us everything we needed.

Something significant happened in Woody's spiritual life that last week.

Though his muscles were gone, he could still lock his joints and attain a rigidity of his arms and legs so that I would have to tell him to relax in order to bend his limbs and turn him.

Four nights before his death, Woody was extremely sick. The next morning he wanted the talk board and spelled out that indeed we hadn't known what God had in store for us—but that we had all accepted it.

"I want to thank you and Danny," he added, "for taking care of me."

"No, Woody," I said. "We thank you for allowing us to care for you—and I know there is a special place in heaven waiting for you."

The next time I had to turn him, he was completely relaxed. His arms and legs were limber. It was as if he had completed the transition of rededication and was ready for the final transition from life to death.

I felt that he would not actually die, but would be reborn into a new and better life.

From that moment, his eyes glowed until the end.

Dr. Lampley returned on Saturday and came immediately to see Woody. Woody was thrilled that he was back; they were such good friends. My mother and father came in, and Woody wanted his talk board. He spelled out that he loved my father, my mother, and all of us very dearly. He wanted us to know that, and he seemed to rest a little better after he told us.

He got a cramp in his foot, and I worked it out.

Before I left that night, I had a feeling he was very near the end. His respiration was down, yet he was coherent enough to talk on the board.

Betty Stevenson's son, whom she hadn't seen in some time, came home to visit, and she had the night off. Dan asked a friend, a young nurse, to stay with him to keep him awake that night, and he insisted that I go home and rest.

I kissed Woody and walked out of the hospital with the feeling that I would never see him alive again.

I went home, laid out my clothes for the next day, and went to bed.

The next morning—Sunday, November 23, 1975—the telephone rang at 7:30. It was Dan.

"Mom," he said, "I think you'd better come back to the hospital now."

I knew that Woody was dead.

"All right," I said. "I'll come immediately."

"No," Dan's voice was firm. "I'm sending Dale for you."

"I'm all right," I said. "I can drive."

"Mom, you don't understand," Dan said. "There is the most beautiful snow I've ever seen."